Conflicted Health Care

Conflicted Health Care

Professionalism and Caring in an Urban Hospital

Ester Carolina Apesoa-Varano
and
Charles S. Varano

VANDERBILT UNIVERSITY PRESS • *Nashville*

© 2014 by Vanderbilt University Press
Nashville, Tennessee 37235
All rights reserved
First printing 2014

Chapter 6, "Crossing the Line," was previously published in a
different form: Apesoa-Varano, Ester Carolina. "Interprofessional
Conflict and Repair: A Study of Boundary Work in the Hospital."
Sociological Perspectives 56, no. 3 (2013): 327–49.

This book is printed on acid-free paper.
Manufactured in the United States of America

Library of Congress Cataloging-in-Publication Data on file
LC control number 2014007694
LC classification number RA972
Dewey class number 362.11068'3—dc23

ISBN 978-0-8265-2008-1 (cloth)
ISBN 978-0-8265-2009-8 (paperback)
ISBN 978-0-8265-2010-4 (ebook)

For Sofia, Ellah, Magali, and Liam

Contents

Acknowledgments

This book culminates years of our ongoing collaboration and shared interests as ethnographers and sociologists. It builds on and reexamines extensive qualitative research that Carolina Apesoa-Varano conducted: she was responsible for the project's conception, design, data collection, and analysis, while Charles Varano provided constant feedback in the form of theoretical and analytical suggestions. We decided to coauthor this book because it reflects how much our personal and professional lives intersect, but because we are at different stages in our academic careers, we each took charge of the manuscript at different stages. Carolina produced its early drafts, with editing from Charles, and Charles handled the final rewrite, with editing and further revisions from Carolina. Both of us actively engaged in refining the analysis and developing the interpretations and theoretical understanding we present in this book.

Given the nature of our collaboration, we struggled with how to achieve an appropriate authorial voice throughout the text. Although the first-person plural pronoun "we" best reflects our collective engagement in the analytical process and our shared interpretation of the data's meaning and theoretical relevance, we have decided to use the first-person singular pronoun "I" throughout the text because Carolina was the only participant observer in the field and this best reflects the ethnographer's voice.

We would like to thank all the hospital practitioners who graciously donated their time outside of work to participate in the research interviews. We also appreciate the practitioners who allowed Carolina to follow them day in and day out, through thick and thin, so that we could learn firsthand what they do for a living. They welcomed Carolina into their world, shared their experiences, and showed her what work and life is in a hospital. In the same light, we want to extend our appreciation to all the administrative staff, managers, and supervisors who helped Carolina maneuver through the bureaucracy of the hospital, introduced her to important contacts, and provided necessary information. Last but not least, we would like to thank the many patients who allowed Carolina into their rooms during the most intimate of moments. Some of them, recovering quickly from their ill-nesses or injuries, were on good terms with life when they left the hospital; others were confined to hospital care for long, long periods of time. Many of them passed away with family by their side; others were not so lucky, and the practitioners who cared for them were the closest they had to friends or family.

This book would not have been possible without the faculty and institu-tional support Carolina received from the Department of Sociology at the University of California, Davis, especially from 2004 to 2008. The Office of Graduate Studies, the Department of Sociology, and the Labor and Employ-ment Research Fund of the University of California Office of the President provided generous financial support to Carolina during the initial writing of the manuscript. Our deepest gratitude goes to Vicki Smith, who me-ticulously read numerous early drafts of the manuscript, offered detailed comments, and closely edited what must have seemed like mind-numbing prose. We also wish to thank Carole Joffe, Ming-Cheng Lo, Beth Bechky, and Drew Halfmann, who all offered invaluable feedback and saw "the for-est for the trees" during this phase of manuscript preparation. At the Uni-versity of Colorado, Boulder, thanks to Martha Gimenez for her intellectual guidance and close friendship and Jane Menken and Tom Mayer for their expertise and encouragement. Bob Kloss and Dean Dorn at California State University, Sacramento, also deserve special thanks: Bob started Carolina down the road of researching nursing for her master's thesis, while Dean read through a late draft of the book and offered useful comments on every chapter. Other colleagues also lent their support through the latter stages of this project, including Heather Young, Judith Barker, Ladson Hinton, Sergio Aguilar-Gaxiola, Stuart Henderson, Jud Landis, and especially Anita Kando, who, with admirable patience and diligence, transcribed countless hours of interviews.

We could not have been more fortunate than to have Michael Ames, of Vanderbilt University Press, as our editor for this book. Michael saw some promise in an early draft of this work and steered us critically yet patiently through the revision process. We greatly appreciate copyeditor Peg Duthie for her careful work clarifying our muddled prose and catching numerous mistakes throughout the manuscript. We also want to thank the Vanderbilt

University Press editorial board, as well as the outside reviewers whose extensive comments alerted us to relevant literature, helped us avoid errors at various points, and guided us in writing a more coherent book.

Finally, we would like to thank Nidia and David Apesoa, Carolina's parents. Nidia served as a pediatrician among the urban poor of Argentina for many years, and we have always been inspired by her personal selflessness and professional commitment to health—something we also found among the practitioners in this hospital. Both she and David offered countless hours of their time to help with childcare, as our children were all born during the research and writing of this book. Sofia Leonor and Ellah Rose both arrived as Carolina worked on the initial drafts, while our twins, Magali Grace and Liam Joseph, joined us during the final year of manuscript revisions.

Introduction

"CODE BLUE, code blue, unit 3, code blue, code blue, unit 3," the speaker system blared, as Mike rushed into a patient's room in disbelief.

"Mike," a clerk yelled, "your guy in 34, he's coding!"

Mike was a competent and pleasant nurse who had worked on the floor for over ten years. Today he was looking after five patients, and among them was a seventy-year-old man who had been admitted through the emergency room in the early morning hours with cardiac symptoms. The patient had seemed stable throughout the morning and was "hooked up" so that his heart rate could be constantly monitored at the nurse's station in case of emergency. We had an emergency.

The patient appeared to be asleep as Mike loudly called out his name. After moving his face near the man's mouth to feel if he was breathing, Mike began rubbing the patient's chest around the heart area. A group of doctors, another nurse, a respiratory therapist, and a pharmacist stormed into the room. Mike placed his finger on the man's neck—"no breathing, no pulse." With everyone hovering over the patient, there was loud yelling, with some people calling for medications and others giving instructions ("get the pads!"). People were moving fast and someone ran out to the supply room.

"Everybody calm down," a physician ordered. "Everyone out of this room except you, you, and you!" The junior residents and interns huddled outside by the door, listening and peering in. Four people remained in the room, disagreeing about one thing or another as they worked on the patient.

After what seemed like a few minutes had passed, Mike sighed, "He's back. He's back, okay, okay," and things started to settle down. At the door, people whispered anxiously to one another. A resident physician, visibly distraught, said to one of the nurses, "I was working on him—that's wrong to kick us out—I'm part of the team." Nodding, the nurse patted her on the back as the patient was wheeled from the room.

Mike kept a close eye on the patient as this took place, and then said to a nurse standing nearby, "Teresa, I'm going up to the OR. Can you watch my other guys?" A little later, as he quietly walked back to the unit, Mike seemed exhausted. Upon entering the room the patient had been in, he saw a social worker gently speaking to a crying woman, with her hand on the woman's shoulder—the woman was the daughter of Mike's patient, and she had just been informed of the incident. Mike tried to comfort the worried daughter, who kept asking if her father would be okay.

It was a strange feeling on the floor: everyone seemed a little tense, yet everything seemed like business as usual. Later that afternoon in the break room, the nurse manager debriefed some junior residents, a social worker, and the nurses who were present. "What happened today was traumatic and that's why I think it is important to talk about it," the nurse manager explained. "I was told people were yelled out of the room and stuff. . . . We are all professionals and we need to work together to handle these situations better."

The social worker insisted that it was unacceptable that family had not been called and that no one "had paid enough attention to notice that the daughter was outside the room when all of this was happening." In a disapproving tone, she continued, "Doctors need to do their job as anyone else in handling things the way they need to be handled."

Mike interjected, "The problem was that everybody was calling the shots," and the room fell silent.

"Well, who was the one in charge of you guys?" the nurse manager asked the physicians.

"But that's not the issue," one of the nurses pleaded. "We know that the doctors are leading the code, but we're all trying to do our jobs because we care about our patients."

A speech therapist who had been sitting quietly in the back of the room said, "Oh come on, guys. This happens all the time."

"But you were not involved this time," the nurse manager said, exasperated.

"But I was last week," the speech therapist replied, "when we had that other situation, remember?"

The atmosphere in the room became increasingly tense, with people shaking their heads or rolling their eyes. As the discussion continued, the social worker stated, "Whatever our differences, we are all here for a reason, and patients depend on us, so . . ."

"Yes," Mike agreed. "It's not about anyone wanting something bad to happen to our patients, but if we are a team, then we need to work that way."

The physicians in the room were noticeably silent through most of the meeting. Eventually, one of the residents said, "Well, you guys have to run things by us and not just assume—"

The nurse manager interrupted the resident, saying, "Look, we are really busy people, and like I said, we're all professionals. Doctors have to do their part to respect everyone else, and that is not what happened today." In a firm voice, she continued: "Let's make sure we communicate as professionals with respect. You know, we all care about our patients—if we didn't, we would be making more money somewhere else." And with that, people started leaving the room to get back to work—to keep working with each other.

"Code blue"—no other phrase creates such an adrenaline rush in hospital staff. It also captures the tension between the codes of professionalism and caring that characterize the modern hospital, medical work, and health care. We often talk of how much we want health-care practitioners to be caring professionals—empathetic and competent, emotionally engaged and technically savvy. Unfortunately, our ideals of what makes a caring professional are grounded on assumptions that are frequently hard to reconcile, particularly for those on the floor facing workplace pressures, organizational bureaucracy, and market imperatives.[1] The vignette above surely reflects the stress of trying to save lives, but it also characterizes the struggle to bridge these ideals. Health workers with diverse professional training and knowledge must act cooperatively—yet, how can they, with everybody "calling the shots"? In the occupational hierarchy of health care, physicians occupy the top of the totem pole. Yet, as this vignette under-scores, they face other practitioners whose sense of professionalism fre-quently evokes challenges to the authority vested within this occupational hierarchy. While practitioners "all care about our patients—if we didn't, we would be making more money somewhere else," the fact remains that "car-ing" means different things to different groups, and it frequently collides head-on with professional interests and organizational constraints. This book explores the relationship between professionalism and caring among five different groups of practitioners in a large urban teaching hospital, how they negotiate interoccupational relations and "teamwork," and how they grapple with the ideal of caring as health-care professionals.

For decades now, popular culture has dramatized the hospital, blending a skeptical if not cynical air with a romanticized view of the work of health-care practitioners. While these fictional portrayals may reinforce the es-teem of those working in health care, they have also likely nurtured our collective ambivalence about whether these practitioners actually merit the social and economic perks they receive—particularly physicians.[2] The heady triumphs of Drs. James Kildare and Ben Casey have been eclipsed by the troubled personal and professional relationships of *Grey's Anatomy* and *House*. Yet, at least in popular culture, the embattled individual health-care worker has remained a heroic foe of the medical establishment, in depic-tions from the 1960s to the present.

Some important scholarly studies have provided systematic accounts of health-care practitioners in the hospital, and we know a good deal about the hospital from an organizational point of view—how it has adapted to the increasing rationalization of services and profit-making pressures in the context of managed care.[3] We also know quite a bit about two ma-jor practitioner groups in the hospital, physicians and nurses. Still, we are less familiar with the daily experiences and perspectives of a wide range of health-care workers, separated by job title, training, and experience but unified by their collective work and ideals. Health-care delivery is a unique milieu in which occupational groups are, by training and tempera-ment, highly autonomous, yet by organizational necessity mutually inter-dependent. What happens when the occupational status hierarchy makes it difficult for health-care workers to live up to their professional aspirations and caring ideals?

This book documents how this status hierarchy, in the context of increasing patient loads and limited time, challenges conventional norms of professionalism while leaving the ideal of caring a figment of its popular and nostalgic image. In the words of a senior physician, "I really appreciate my clinic hours away from Hospital General because I can spend more time with each patient, rather than having to watch the clock."[4] A nurse put it bluntly: "The caring stuff comes later, and if you can do it, fine, but otherwise it is not a priority." How are we to understand these laments, coming as they do from people who have entered fields that in both popular and occupational cultures have elevated caring to a calling? Most analyses of professions have glossed over the caring activities that characterize much professional work, particularly health practitioners' work at the bedside. The scholarship on professions and care work are rarely connected, whereas this book bridges the divide.[5] Specifically, I consider how all these groups struggle to uphold an ideal of caring—in discourse and in practice—in the midst of an occupational hierarchy, organizational factors, and professional norms that render caring activities less important and devalued relative to medical interventions associated with curing.

Though my primary concern with the balancing act of professionalism and caring is largely academic, I also share the concerns of anyone who has spent time in a hospital as a patient or family member of a patient. Certainly we all hope that those who might attend to us or our loved ones will be at their professional best, and that they will care for us in ways that console our fears and preserve our dignity as humans (especially when we are most fragile). These concerns have been heightened in the context of the ongoing crisis of health-care costs and provision in the United States (the 2010 Patient Protection and Affordable Care Act notwithstanding). Likewise, a series of Institute of Medicine reports (including a 2010 report on nursing) testifies to the ongoing problems of health care in the United States and the "strong medicine" necessary to remedy these organizational ills.[6] Lest one assume that the tension between professionalism and caring afflicts only those who visit a hospital in an HMO-market-based health-care system (i.e., in the United States), one need only glance at the recent Mid Staffordshire scandal in England's National Health System. An independent inquiry chaired by Robert Francis, QC (Queen's Counsel), uncovered disturbing details, summed up by reporter Oliver Wright as "catastrophic failures [that] started at the patients' bedside but reached up, through the Byzantine hierarchy of the NHS, to [the] heart of Government. From the nurses who left patients in excrement-soiled bed clothes to the managers who only wanted 'good' news, to the Health Secretaries obsessed with financial targets, no-one emerges with credit from the Mid Staffordshire scandal."[7] Indeed, one could view conflicted health care as epitomizing a shriveling social contract, as well as the global austerity policies of our time.

As I have written this book for a general audience, I will limit academic references in the body of the text to those most relevant to my arguments. For those who wish to pursue the broader scholarship that informs my analysis, I have placed the references to those sources in the endnotes. A preliminary review, however, is necessary at this point to provide the framework for my arguments through the rest of this book.

In exploring the tension between professionalism and caring ethnographically, I adopt an interactionist perspective, where the hospital is seen as a negotiated social order. This approach derives from the work of Erving Goffman on total institutions and William Caudill on mental hospitals.[8] Yet, within this tradition, Anselm Strauss's work remains the most extensive body of theorizing on hospitals and medical work.[9] The hospital, Strauss argues, is a negotiated order because it entails interactions that do not "occur by chance, but are patterned."[10] Because formal rules and mandates guiding patient treatment are too generalized, practitioners must negotiate how a particular patient ought to be treated. For Strauss, negotiations become increasingly complex because members of various occupational fields hold different views not only about patient treatment and the meaning of illness and recovery but also about whose judgment is more legitimate, what type of judgment is being applied, and whether they view each other as professionals or not. This "diversity of purpose affects the institution's division of labor," not only in terms of which task each group is expected to perform but also how each group goes about accomplishing it on a daily basis.[11] Most importantly, Strauss contends that the hierarchical position of the practitioners, their ideology, and the structure of ward relationships are the most influential factors shaping the nature and outcome of routine negotiations on the hospital floor.

Within this negotiated order, professional roles are not only reproduced but also challenged as ambiguities in the division of labor and in patient conditions become apparent. It is at these points (which occur more frequently than we generally assume) that what Andrew Abbott calls "jurisdictional disputes" emerge and are resolved—albeit only partially and temporarily. Abbott contends that jurisdictional struggles reflect attempts to control arenas of work, and that the most consequential professional struggles occur over the assertion of competence and theoretical knowledge about how a specific phenomenon works and how a profession is able to effectively resolve an identified problem.[12] In Hospital General, these disputes are mediated by an emphasis on "teamwork," whereby coordination of roles and unity of purpose are supposed to transcend occupational differences and authority relations. Despite its widespread appeal, however, the teamwork ideal is more an *ideology* in managing labor, given how the occupational hierarchy routinely undermines professional sentiments and aspirations.[13] Personal conflicts are endemic in large organizational settings and I do not wish to exaggerate their frequency or importance in this book. I am arguing, however, that the conflicts and disagreements I document here are structural in nature, and not merely the result of personality, inclination, or malice. They emerge from how the authority structure in Hospital General (and arguably in every hospital in the United States and abroad) rests on occupational claims to knowledge that are contested on a daily basis.

Scholars of care work in post-industrial society provide the other important piece of the complex story told in this book. Theorizing and research on caring have focused on institutions from the family and schools to the workplace in general and health care in particular, and feminist scholars have long argued that caring and care work are devalued, both in terms of remuneration and social status.[14] In *The Invisible Heart*, feminist economist Nancy Folbre makes a compelling case for how a competitive market economy inadequately provides the care necessary for social well-being and progress, and she eloquently argues that we have a collective (not just women's) responsibility to provide it to one another. Yet, in Hospital General, although caring meant different things to different groups, it was still subordinate to a dominant cure orientation based in biomedical science and intervention. Even if one were to view a "caring practitioner" as someone doing their job to the best of their ability—a claim made by many practitioners, especially physicians—they still unanimously held that emotive caring was not part of that job. In *Beyond Caring*, Daniel Chambliss argues persuasively that nurses utilize caring as an occupational strategy to advance their interests and raise their status, especially vis-à-vis physicians. While the nurses in Hospital General espoused the importance of emotive caring in treating patients, they hardly had the time to deploy this strategy, much less accrue any advantages or benefits from it, *nor did they seem to want to.* The nurses I spoke with (along with nursing students I interviewed a few years ago) sought to reconcile biomedical knowledge and skills with emotive caring in the practice of nursing.[15] It seems as though evoking the importance of emotive caring has been abandoned as a preferred occupational strategy, even though it still exacts a symbolic—and psychic—toll in the hearts and minds of nurses and other practitioners alike.

This issue has been amplified in the past decade by key scholars of nursing. Having reviewed research studies on the social organization of nursing work from 1993 to 2003, Davina Allen argues that nurses have "little to gain by continuing to pursue an agenda of holistic patient care based on emotional intimacy" and should instead embrace their role as health care mediators with patients and staff.[16] Likewise, as Sioban Nelson and Suzanne Gordon argue in *The Complexities of Care*, nurses still cling to an ideal of emotive caring as part of their occupational mandate, even though they regularly demonstrate their knowledge and medical skills in treating patients.[17] For Nelson and Gordon, nursing and nurses would be better served were they to embrace and emphasize their medical knowledge and skills in caring for patients and achieving better health outcomes. Yet, though these skills (including mediation skills) are evident in their daily routines, this way of framing the work of nurses and other practitioners overlooks the skills associated with emotive caring—skills that are arguably as difficult to master as the medical skills, and arguably as important to patient well-being and health outcomes. For instance, in *Deciding Who Lives*, Renee Anspach shows how nurses and physicians in two neonatal intensive care units arrive at different judgments because their working conditions generate different sources of knowledge about the condition of seriously ill infants. Specifically, because physicians have far less contact with patients, they are more invested in the "objective" data supplied by technology and measurement, whereas nurses, because they spend far more time with these children, come to rely more on the "subjective" interactional cues that "are rarely entered into patients' charts systematically" and thus "cannot be validated as prognostic signs."[18] Consequently, the knowledge derived from emotive caring—as well, I would argue, the skills involved in providing it— are devalued in the hospital setting and rejected in favor of the knowledge and skills associated with curative intervention, even if such interventions might be more thoughtfully arrived at and successfully conducted were they informed by emotive caring. Perhaps abandoning the holistic caring mandate may be premature.

In Hospital General, I found that emotive caring is not supported except as an ideal (like teamwork) that obscured organizational neglect and therefore rendered individual caring as virtuous and even heroic. And though some occupations enjoy more structured time to provide emotive caring (e.g., occupational, physical, and speech [OPS] therapists and social workers), the fact remains that it is an aspect of hospital work that nobody has time for and everybody subordinates to curative interventions.[19] As we will see in the case of OPS therapists, only when emotive caring is coupled with curative interventions and health outcomes based in biomedical science does it engender a positive valuation. Conversely, occupations that consider it a primary aspect of their labor such as social work remain notably marginal in the hospital milieu.

In this context, caring and professionalism become alienated from one another in the conflicted health care at Hospital General. While practitioners still refer to caring as a strategy, it is not necessarily to prevail in interoccupational conflicts, but rather to resist the most inhumane aspects of health care, as well as to advance or defend different versions of professional caring.[20] Here, ideology is not exclusively a symbolic weapon deployed in organizational battle, for the sake of defending or advancing a narrow self-interest; rather, ideology is also a blueprint of sorts, for a social order that might yield more rewards for more people to enjoy at less physical, emotional, and psychic cost.[21] It is in this advocacy sense of the term "ideology" that I also heard practitioners express what it was like to practice emotive caring with patients—and each other.

Hospital General

Hospital General is an intimidating place. It is a sprawling architectural maze, and everyone working there seems to move through its endless corridors with an aura of certainty and belonging. By contrast, patients and their families wander about, trying to figure out where they are going, some carrying flowers or a cup of coffee, some with somber faces, some crying, and some smiling and seemingly reassured.

Hospital General used to be a county hospital until the early 1970s, when a university seeking to expand its medical school acquired the hospital as a "lab" for medical students and residents to practice and develop clinical skills. Since then, it has become a major training institution not only for medical residents but also for those training in other occupations, such as nursing, social work, respiratory therapy, and rehabilitation therapy. The hospital is well known in the region, especially for the quality of the practitioners it recruits at various levels of patient care. Hospital General also boasts a highly trained staff of registered nurses, and its various medical programs and specialties have garnered national acclaim over the years.

The campus has three main areas, each corresponding to a different age or stage of the hospital. The central hospital is housed in the original five-story building. Even though there are still some units functioning there, most of it is occupied by different labs, a blood bank, and administrative and academic offices. Some of the patient units were moved to newer areas of Hospital General, because the original wards were found unsuitable for patient care and they remain empty; one cannot help imagining an abandoned ghost town while walking through them. This part of the hospital is pretty decrepit, and the units that still function there (i.e., neurosurgery and cardio step-down) are old, dark, crowded, and neither patient- nor worker-friendly. For example, the nurses' break rooms and bathrooms are inadequate, the medication rooms are small, the nurses' stations are crowded, the hallways are narrow, and the tiny patient rooms make it hard to maneuver if there are two patients and more than two practitioners in them.

A newer building, constructed as an addition to the central hospital, contains the regular medical-surgical floors, all the intensive care units (ICUs), the post-anesthesia unit, and the operating rooms. It is a seven-story building that is a bit more modern-looking (e.g., with better lighting and windows, and newer paint) than the central hospital, and the layout of the units is worker-friendlier. The medical-surgical units in this section form a rectangle, with the patient rooms around the periphery. In the center, there is a nurses' station, along with break rooms, the nurse manager's office, a nutrition room, a supply room, a medication room, and a cleaning/storage room.

The ICUs vary in functionality and organization, but they all have glass-encased, single-occupancy rooms where patients can be observed from any place at the nurses' station. In the ICUs, the circulation and movement of nurses and other staff is more confined, since patients are supposed to get individual care and close monitoring. Nurses spend most of their time at small tables outside the glass encasements, where they can observe monitors displaying a patient's vital signs (such as heart rate, pulse, and oxygenation); the tables hold the patients' charts, drinks, and medications, and whatever else might be needed for their care. These floors, though an improvement over the main building, seem invariably worn out and hardly more inviting.

The nicest and most recent addition to the hospital is a twelve-story building that features wide hallways, wood wall details, artwork, and large patient rooms with large windows and modern decor. This building has more than one nurses' station, as well as large break rooms, physicians' lounges and sleep/rest rooms, large staff bathrooms, a few nutrition rooms, ample storage and supply rooms, large medication rooms, and a medica-tion dispensing machine in each nurses' station. It also has a conference room and internal elevators for staff such as food service and maintenance. Interestingly, there is a social hierarchy expressed in the location of units in this building. For example, the orthopedics unit, with its busy money-making surgeries, is located on the highest floor, which offers the best views of the city, the surrounding mountains, and the occasionally exhilarating, action-filled moments when the medical helicopter approaches and lands on the building terrace. This unit also has several VIP rooms (usually large corner rooms with huge glass windows, chairs, a table, and other ameni-ties) for individual patients who garner preferential treatment. The cancer unit, tightly administered by an old-school nurse manager, is on an upper floor that still enjoys some nice views and has ample accommodations for staff but no VIP patient rooms. As a last example, the labor and delivery unit has a spacious reception entrance, a triage area, and one small OR, but no VIP rooms. The rooms generally overlook the roof of the lower sides of the building, and the nurses have a tiny break room where only four of them can sit at any one time. This unit has a small nutrition room, only one nurse's station, and one medication and supply room. The hierarchy of medical specialties and units seems to be reflected in their floor location within Hospital General.

These three buildings are connected by long and seemingly endless hallways with several sets of elevators and stairs. Walking through these hallways, one finds countless doors that always seem locked and through which no one enters or departs, leaving one to wonder what might be going on behind them. The most startling yet intriguing part of the hospital is the underground floor, where one can find everyone and everything that is marginal, invisible, or unwanted; it is the repository of all the human and nonhuman waste that the hospital produces. Here, too, there is a hierarchy, of the cook, the cleaner, and the laundry worker. The basement floor is also where disabled people from the community work, cleaning cafeteria tables or helping in the kitchen as part of a work program. Interestingly, the only cafeteria in the whole hospital is located here, along with the home departments of the OPS therapy services, some conference rooms, and some resident and intern locker rooms. This is basically the guts of the hospital, with cement floors, grey and off-white walls, overhead pipes, and a maze-like quality. One can easily get lost in this area and come out smelling like ultra-deep-fried fish and chips.

Finally, there are many adjacent buildings, housing clinics, administrative and academic offices, storage units, a police station, pathology labs, and the morgue. These buildings, in addition to the actual inpatient hospital I have described above, constitute a vast medical complex.

During the research period, many important things happened in Hospital General, and a few of these deserve a brief mention. Like many teaching hospitals in the country, Hospital General struggled to maintain adequate physician staffing while respecting the eighty-hour limit on residents' workweeks. The emergency flight program was shut down because of budget cuts; most of the nurses employed by the program did not lose their jobs, since they were reassigned in-house, but the situation was highly conflictive. Compounding this, the nursing staff in the OR was very unhappy with a new manager, which created a highly volatile working environment and a problem for nursing administration. The nurses' union began negotiations about numerous issues that eventually stalled and led to a strike vote. Likewise, the respiratory therapy department hired a new manager who was set on addressing its "culture of complacency" and poor professionalism, which caused dissension among its staff. To complicate matters further, there were two strikes by different groups of employees in maintenance and transportation (including cooks, janitors, and drivers), which kept the hospital administration busy with bargaining. Yet, on a positive note, the hospital administration began a multi-million-dollar plan to vastly improve its core services, and it inaugurated a state-of-the-art vascular clinic that has become renowned among the few in the country.

Studying Hospital General

The research for this book combines ethnographic data (participant observation) and in-depth interviews. During the initial period of observation (2004–2005), I conducted 110 interviews with practitioners working in the hospital, each varying in length from one and a half to three hours. Specifically, the sample is composed of twenty-one medical doctors, thirty registered nurses, twenty-one respiratory therapists, twenty medical social workers, and eighteen occupational, physical, and speech therapists.[22] While much research has been conducted on physicians and nurses, and some on social workers, the other two groups remain virtually unexplored, and that is partly why they were included in this project. I also selected these five groups because: (1) they constitute a unique case study of professionals *interacting with one another*, which I wanted to analyze, given that previous research has focused on physician-nurse and professional-client relationships, (2) these are the primary occupational groups *caring for* patients, and (3) their interactions reveal a great deal about the *contested nature* of professionalism and caring in the modern hospital.[23]

I also conducted 2,700 hours of participant observation, covering twelve-hour shifts four to five days a week in a variety of units from 2004 to 2005. I continued more focused observations (over five hundred hours) through 2006–2007 by visiting units and talking to practitioners about issues that required further clarity or elaboration. I observed practitioners at work in the operating room, postoperative recovery unit, adult medical-surgical floors, orthopedics unit, pediatric unit, labor and delivery unit, and adult and pediatric intensive care units. In addition, I spent some time in the home departments of each occupation, where I had many conversations with practitioners during breaks or at the beginning or end of their shifts.

Ethnographic research in a large teaching hospital is not easy, first and foremost because of the difficulties one faces in obtaining access: Hospital General is a highly guarded and protective institution, and the many legal and regulatory guidelines make the process of gaining entrée even more daunting. I made many contacts at different levels of the institution and across occupational groups, repeatedly explaining the project and its potential contributions to practitioners, the hospital, and related fields of scholarship. After many face-to-face meetings, e-mails, phone calls, and

formal letters, and after working through bureaucratic red tape, I began my
first shift of observations and initial interviews in the fall of 2004.

Readers of this book may wonder if a teaching hospital is representative of other private and public hospitals. A teaching hospital, however, is
perhaps the best site to learn about professionalism and caring, and about
organizational models such as team delivery of health services. Because
of the educational, training, and mentoring goals of the teaching hospital,
professionalism and caring are central to its mission and thus heavily emphasized. If these are contentious or problematic issues in this setting, then
they are likely even more so in for-profit or nonteaching hospitals, where
organizational hierarchies are more demarcated and entrenched and where
the organizational culture is perhaps less vested in such lofty goals in the
context of managed care. I believe there is much we can learn and ask about
professionalism and caring in the teaching hospital that is very relevant to
other hospital settings. In any event, I leave it to readers to arrive at their
own judgments, based on the story I tell of Hospital General and their own
hospital experiences.

A final vignette highlights the chapter topics to follow. As a husband
and his pregnant wife are ushered into one of the triage rooms in Labor
and Delivery, one of the nurses waves me over to observe. After the couple
generously approves of my presence, a nursing student begins taking vital
signs (blood pressure, heart rate, temperature) while the senior nurse asks
the woman some questions: "How far along are you? How much bleeding do you think you've had—enough to soak a pad, or just spotting? How
many days have you noticed this? Have you experienced any cramping?
Any contractions?" Clearly both the wife and the husband are concerned,
and they seem increasingly so as the nurse questions them about the pregnancy. As the nursing student rolls in an ultrasound machine and begins
untangling the cords, swinging them over the bed to reach an electrical
outlet, the senior nurse tries to be reassuring: "What you're experiencing
could be nothing. Some women have bleeding at this stage of pregnancy,"
she says. "Just as long as you're not bleeding a lot over many days and you're
not experiencing contractions. But we're going to have the doctor come in
and check to make sure everything is okay, and we have that heartbeat, so
try not to worry."

Try not to worry? Even I was worried as we stepped outside to wait
for the physician. But what I call the "professional self" is certainly reas-

suring, especially to patients who are anything but reassured by their situation. In Chapter 1, I introduce each occupation as expressed through interviews with physicians, nurses, OPS therapists, respiratory therapists, and social workers. I prefer the term "professional self" to "professional identity" because it highlights how professionalism is socially constructed by members of an occupation in relation to other occupations. Yet I do not mean to ignore how professionalism involves ideological claims on the part of occupations seeking to advance or defend their interests in and across organizational settings as Magali Sarfatti Larson argued in *The Rise of Professionalism*. Depending on their position in Hospital General's status hierarchy and division of labor, practitioners view professionalism differently in terms of knowledge, norms, and teamwork.[24] As I show in Chapter 2, this professional self is routinely challenged on the floor in interoccupational struggles among differently ranked practitioners. I explore these struggles in the context of a teamwork ideal that is formally promoted by the hospital and embraced by practitioners but ultimately heightens occupational differences rather than alleviating them.

As we wait for the physician, I can only imagine how the pregnant woman and her husband must feel, and what has seemed like minutes to me must seem like hours to them. But waiting for another practitioner is common in Hospital General, and something that frequently taxes the patience and ideals of practitioners as well as patients, especially the caring ideal. The caring ideal is complex, but it can be usefully distinguished by whether practitioners speak of "caring *about*" or "caring *for*" patients as well as one another. Every practitioner referred to caring *about* patients insofar as they sought to perform their job as best they could. Yet when practitioners spoke of caring *for* patients, the ideal of caring became harder to uphold, as the practices associated with emotive caring (e.g., interacting with patients at an emotional level, spending time with patients, and consoling patients who are anxious, confused, angry, or in pain) ranked second to the cure orientation that dominates work in Hospital General. Consequently, as I argue in Chapter 3, caring becomes cast as an individual virtue rather than an organizationally supported aspect of health care. Just as teamwork fails to transcend the status hierarchy in Hospital General, so too does caring fall short, as I show in Chapter 4. In this context, a caring ideology is promoted by hospital administration in managing labor, particularly that of nurses, but I also argue that caring can be understood as a form of resistance to the objectification of patients at the bedside and the growing specter of practitioner exploitation. Like in any other complex organization, practitioners faced working conditions that challenged their professional and caring ideals, and I consider how they viewed these problems in Chapter 5, where I show how the most serious problems facing practitioners, specifically time and people, are social problems that involve negotiating relationships—whether it is with patients, other practitioners, or hospital administrators. This chapter serves to bridge my analysis in the previous chapters with those to follow, as it outlines the working conditions that practitioners must navigate in their struggle to resolve the tensions between professionalism and caring.

When the physician arrives, he appears distracted, as if his body is in the room but his mind is elsewhere. At this point of the pregnancy, it is necessary to use an intravaginal ultrasound to confirm the heartbeat of the fetus, so I back into a corner of the room to afford the woman as much privacy as possible. Not so the physician, senior nurse, and nursing student, who all crowd as closely as possible around the woman. After several minutes of prodding and poking, much to the discomfort of the woman—lying exposed to all—it becomes apparent that the physician is finding it difficult to pinpoint the precise location of the heartbeat.

Ever so gently, the senior nurse reaches over to the monitor and points it out to the physician and nursing student. "Ah yes," the physician says. "Here we go, a steady heartbeat." Never once does he acknowledge that he had trouble identifying the heartbeat, nor does he thank the nurse who did (though, after he leaves, the woman and her husband thank her profusely).

This interaction illustrates one of two ways that a balance between professionalism and caring might be struck. In Chapter 6, I explore how practitioners frequently cross into each other's domains of practice or expertise and in many cases demonstrate knowledge or insight that exceeds that of higher-status practitioners. Though this "boundary work" is ultimately motivated by how deeply practitioners care about their patients in the context of organizational problems—thus constituting an informal system of teamwork that might symbolically bridge professionalism and caring—it ultimately reproduces the occupational hierarchy and the devaluation of caring. I then consider a second way that practitioners balance professionalism and caring in Chapter 7 by showing how their views toward unions underscore the ideological nature of both. Here, unionism is the counterpoint to teamwork, because it can unite practitioners, but only in the context of an even more intractable division between those who support and those who oppose unions.

As everyone leaves the room, the physician tells the woman that she was right to ask to be admitted: "Don't be afraid to call any time you think something's not right. That's what we're here for." The senior nurse chimes in: "There's no guarantee with pregnancy, but we're here to take care of you when you need us. The attending physician will drop in to check on you shortly." The nursing student smiles as she leaves the room, and I sense a bit of relief in the faces of the woman and her husband.

Within the next hour, however, I am surprised to see the husband slowly walk out of the room and look around the hall for a nurse. "Can we leave now," he asks in a tired voice, "or do we have to wait for another doctor to check my wife?" After looking at the woman's chart, the senior nurse tells the man that he can wait for the attending physician if he wants to, but that his wife is cleared to leave. Watching him from the nurses' station, I am struck by the strain and distress pulling at the man's face as he slowly returns to his wife's room, and I wonder where is all the professionalism and caring I had heard so much about. In my concluding chapter, I reconsider possible ways to balance these ideals, and whether, when all is said and done, they are even reconcilable at all.

Chapter 1

The Professional Self

Maybe we are all professionals in different ways.
—ATTENDING PHYSICIAN

W HAT DOES IT MEAN to be a "professional" working among others who also claim this coveted status? To answer this question, I interviewed practitioners at length about what it meant to be a professional in their field. Here, I use the term "professional self" to refer to a set of core aspects that are collectively understood to be characteristic of members of an occupation in general and their role in the hospital. In using the term "self," I wish to encourage readers to view the occupations I introduce in this chapter not as static categories or entities but rather as negotiated roles that are as much a product of one's historically structured position in an organization as the ideological claims made by practitioners to defend or advance their position. As practitioners grappled with what they believed epitomized professionalism in their fields, their views revealed that the professional self is as much a field of conflict among practitioners as it is the answer to life and death for many patients.

The practitioners of each occupation I introduce below all thought of themselves as professionals, though the meaning of the term was subtly different among them in the context of larger occupational issues and their roles in the hospital. Still, in my interviews, three general dimensions of the professional self emerged recurrently across all five groups: (1) knowledge, (2) occupational norms, and (3) teamwork. The hallmark of professional work has always been the degree to which its actors enjoy occupational autonomy and exercise control over the labor process.[1] Their claims to autonomy and control rest on their possession of specialized, "esoteric" knowledge and their ability to abide by occupational norms without direct supervision or oversight. Unlike knowledge and norms, however, team-work is an aspect of professional work that aligns awkwardly with occu-pational claims to autonomy and control over one's labor, for how can one be autonomous and control one's own labor if one must work with other practitioners claiming professional status on a team that is hierarchically structured? Because the teamwork component is difficult to reconcile, it is easily the weakest link of the professional self, highlighting practitioner vulnerability across a terrain of challenges. Rather than smoothing out oc-cupational status rankings, the idea of teamwork actually *heightens* these differences and the tensions arising therein. Therefore, the subheadings I use are intended to evoke the central dilemma facing each group, rather than to offer any definitive characterization.

"Teams" at Hospital General were typically composed of attending physicians (who fulfill clinical, teaching, research, and administrative re-sponsibilities), physicians in training (i.e., fellows and residents), registered nurses, and providers of allied or support services (all licensed), such as social workers, respiratory therapists, and physical, occupational, and speech therapists.[2] Yet the teams did not exist as formal entities created by hospital administrators or occupational directors (except in the case of, say, physicians, who were organized along seniority lines: attending, senior resident, interns, and so on). Rather, the term "team" was used more rhe-torically—or, as Rachael Finn puts it, "discursively"—in referring to the col-lective activities of different specialists and different occupations in serving patients.[3] There were some highly coordinated teams (e.g., operating room teams) and less coordinated teams (e.g., nonspecialized units), and "team members" varied, depending on shift schedules or who was on call to pro-vide specialty services.

Lastly, I found it conspicuously notable that caring was rarely mentioned in my interviews when discussing professionalism. What could arguably be considered a central aspect of professional work—perhaps even one of the strongest defenses of professional privileges and power—seemed a distant and remote concern of practitioners. During my research, it was obvious how much practitioners cared about their patients and their work, but in terms of professionalism—as ideal or ideology—caring clearly ranked well below knowledge and the norms informing its use. This reinforced for me just how much caring has been humbled in the minds of hospital practitioners—even among nurses, for whom it has historically bestowed some degree of status, some measure of respect, and some ideological leverage in relation to physicians and other practitioners.[4] Though a mixed blessing for nurses, who have long struggled for recognition and respect, it was also a troubling sign of just how estranged caring and the professional self were in Hospital General.

The "Good" Doctor

Dr. Whitmore, a woman in her fifties, is a pediatrician. While approachable and unassuming, she also exudes a certain strength and an air of authority. "It's hard to be a good doctor," she told me on numerous occasions. "It's really an art." Often, she reiterated that it is not just a matter of having the necessary clinical skills, but also how the doctor deals with problems and people. "We [doctors] are human," she mused over coffee one afternoon, "even though people think we are perfect. There are professional doctors, and there are unprofessional ones—good and bad apples everywhere." As I spoke with more physicians, it appeared that Dr. Whitmore's views reflected those of her hospital colleagues, which raised more doubts than one might expect.

Physicians have epitomized professionalism both in popular culture and academic scholarship. Yet the physicians I interviewed were engaged in a larger debate that was taking place within the occupation, among medical leaders, and in current research, on the tenuous nature of their medical authority.[5] This concern over authority arose amid controversies during the second half of the twentieth century, when physicians faced public condemnation for lacking ethics or a commitment to the common good.[6] Since then, physician professionalism has met with growing skepticism. As Paul Starr observes, "While Americans express confidence in their own personal physicians, they are more hostile to doctors as a class. The desire to enter medicine as a career is undiminished, but there is great antagonism toward those who do."[7] While the public still holds considerable respect for physicians, the authority of the "all mighty doc" has been increasingly questioned, as calls for second and third opinions attest.

This history was not lost among the physicians I interviewed, a majority of whom thought that "being competent" was central to professionalism.

Their responses, however, were far from simple. For some, competence was not easy to pin down. In the words of Dr. Janis, a surgeon:

> My concern is that there are people that are not competent and don't feel like they are incompetent. . . . They think that what they are doing is competent. I would say that there is a system problem there. The system [occupation] needs to figure out how to define competence. I think that one of the things that is not readily apparent to the nonmedical public is that medicine is by no means a clean, pure science. . . . I can give you a multiple-choice test and say, "Wow, you really know a lot about this fancy pathology, etc." But what is not so easy to test is your ability to apply that at the patient's bedside. It turns out that patients don't present with multiple-choice type questions. With each passing year, it gets harder and harder to weed someone out who is not competent or unprofessional.

When pressed, physicians often equated professionalism to being a "good" doctor. As Dr. Thompson, a cardiologist, explained:

> I guess it would be hard for me to say what that [professionalism] was, except from being a really good physician. A really good physician is somebody who is highly capable with what they do: they can elicit the kind of information they need from the person and then make a decision about what to do and how to determine what they have and how to come up with a good treatment. So [to do] all of that stuff and then do it in a respectful way—that would be my definition of a good physician.

While it was difficult for physicians to agree on the parameters of medical competence and how these might be effectively monitored and enforced, this reflected doubt not over the fundamentals of biomedical knowledge, but rather over how that knowledge should be applied by all hospital physicians. Typically, physicians emphasized their ability to channel complex abstract knowledge into effective intervention techniques to alleviate or cure disease. But ability did not always translate into competence, in light of their descriptions of a "good doctor" as an individual who was not merely technically effective but also *morally* sound. A good deal of symbolic power—and reputation—was at stake when this moral aspect of competence was in doubt, especially among others in the hospital who also identified themselves as professionals.

Affirming their medical competence, then, was only part of the story for physicians, who also spoke of occupational norms in defining a professional self. Dr. Johnson assured me that "professionals like physicians have good manners, have ethical conduct, and have good moral values." In a similar light, another physician explained that a professional physician "is a person that is a 'physician's physician' or a 'gentleman's physician,' where you don't see this [negative or bad] side of the man. . . . They are a true gentleman's gentleman. . . . They're cool, they are natural and likable, and they have a confidence about them. . . . and also they behave themselves in a good manner."

Apart from the gendered nature of this physician's view, professionals were held to normative rules guiding personal conduct and the presentation of self. Physicians considered this normative dimension in the context of a person's moral character, manners, and virtues, including the ability to maintain healthy dose of "confidence" without appearing arrogant—something requiring self-discipline and control. This emphasis on occupational norms made sense particularly in relation to perceptions of physician abuse of power, given their authority in the hospital.[8] Speaking to this issue directly, Dr. Barnes shared the concerns of most physicians I interviewed:

> I define it as a physician acting appropriately . . . that you have
> integrity and honesty. Even when nobody is looking, you want to do
> the right thing. . . . Treating others with kindness and respect. . . .
> And this is a lot to accomplish daily. I would say that most physi-
> cians are not perfect in being this. . . . I think there haven't been
> good examples set in the past because a lot of physicians have had a
> big power trip. . . . We [physicians] have a lot of authority, and then
> we abuse that authority . . . like yelling at residents and being mean
> to patients.

Physicians often found themselves having to reconcile the control and autonomy characteristic of their high-ranking positions with the negative stereotypes of their conduct with other practitioners and patients. Being a professional meant maintaining an uncorrupted self in light of the many external pressures and temptations for self-benefit that those with power and authority frequently face. "You have to be as honest and ethical as the day is long," one physician said with a smile, "even when no one is around." Occupational norms were quite difficult to enforce, given the autonomy physicians enjoy in what they do and how they do it, and the potential abuse of privilege seemed to haunt their professional self.[9] As one of the department chiefs confided, "No physician wants to be told how to behave." Nor do they want their control over their labor challenged. Along with expertise, ethical behavior is central to defending this control.

Physicians also told me that being a professional entailed teamwork. When asked to elaborate, most physicians said that professionalism involved providing good management and direction to other staff regarding patient care. "You have to be able to deal with people," one physician explained, "in a way that your decisions and management are respected." In relation to other practitioners, physicians exercised more authority in deciding protocol for any particular patient—they were the leaders of the team. As one of them put it:

> We must all work together. . . . We are a team—the nurses, the other
> staff, social workers, etc. . . . It is important to get along like a team,
> but we all do different aspects of the puzzle. . . . We all do our little
> part and we [physicians] are the ones who decide on everything,
> and we have to make sure that others [nurses, etc.] know that, but
> they're a really important part of the team.

The professional self had to find its place in a web of highly interrelated groups of practitioners in the hospital. As team leaders, physicians still had to grapple with their reliance on others; they had to recognize the power disparity and frequent antagonisms with other groups on the team while simultaneously establishing rapport with those groups and garnering their support. Getting along with and being part of the team were important, because without the cooperation and good faith of the other groups, working relations among the team members could easily deteriorate, which would then potentially undermine their patients' recovery and ultimately the physicians' authority as good—competent and ethical—leaders.

In light of their reputations as "power trippers," the physicians' professional self revolved around them being *uncorrupted, benevolent leaders,* which required some ideological tinkering in order to integrate competence, occupational norms, and teamwork. Compared to other practitioners, what is noteworthy about the physician professional self is how individualistic it is; as they enact their role, they are far more insulated from the purview and control of others than practitioners in the other groups.[10] Apart from medical review boards and HMO regulations, it is up to the physician to exercise the personal diligence, composure, and self-control necessary to "measure up" to their professional standards. Even the "uncorrupted benevolence" of team leadership evokes a personal character trait rather than any quality that arises in relation to others. Ultimately, this moral individualism is what separates the professional self of physicians from all the other practitioners in Hospital General.

The "Expert" Consultant

Larry Dawson, a man in his early forties, has been a physical therapist for about ten years. He and his colleagues begin each day shift by gathering in the main room, where they receive their assignments and the manager briefly reviews the "load" (schedule of patients) on a whiteboard. After hearing of my interest in professionalism, Larry remarked, "Well, you're in the right place. You know, there's so much talk about being professional these days." He paused. Then, nodding his head, he added, "But really what matters to us is that we are the experts in rehab and we fulfill an important role here [in the hospital]." As we headed to see his first patient, he continued, "I mean, doctors really come to us for our recommendations. They consult with us because we are experts in physiotherapy." Viewing himself as an expert consultant was important to Larry, and I wondered if other OPS therapists thought likewise.

Larry's views had "baggage," both with a small "b" (reflecting floor politics) and a large "B" (reflecting occupational history). OPS therapists emerged as an offshoot of physicians, who delegated less specialized aspects of medical rehabilitation and treatment to them at the turn of the twentieth century. Their initial title as "reconstructive aides" during the years following World War I actually captured the essence of OPS therapists' role in assisting patient recovery alongside nurses and under the supervision of physicians.[11] Like nurses, OPS therapists have historically sought to upgrade the occupation by asserting their ability to use expert knowledge effectively.[12] By the 1970s, OPS therapists could legally provide services outside the hospital, independent of physician supervision. Advancing toward professional autonomy in the early 1980s, OPS therapists were granted the legal right to provide therapy without physician referral.[13] And, most recently, the professional association for physical therapy has moved toward requiring a doctorate for its therapists in clinical practice.

This struggle for independence invariably showed among the OPS therapists I interviewed: they unanimously viewed knowledge as critical to their role as expert consultants to physicians and other groups like nurses.[14] As Melinda, a speech therapist, explained, a professional speech therapist is "someone who is very committed to their profession and stays current on research, new techniques, etc." The therapist "knows well what the patient's needs are . . . and what techniques work best for each type of injury. . . . It's about others like physicians relying on our knowledge and our decisions of what is appropriate for a patient."

For practitioners in the rehabilitation groups, professionalism centered on being clinicians who can identify a biological, physical, or organic basis for a problem and arrive at an appropriate course of treatment or therapy. OPS therapists constructed a professional self by emphasizing the scientific basis of their work, something that allowed them to establish common ground with physicians while pursuing a specialized jurisdiction separate from them. This was not easily achieved, however, as their overzealousness often suggested. When they spoke of their role in making appropriate and crucial recommendations to doctors, they drew a fine distinction in distancing themselves from other groups, like nurses, who worked *for* rather than *with* physicians. As Ryan, one of the physical therapists put it, professional physical therapists "know the body. They can anticipate diagnostically what's going to happen, what they [patients] are going to look like in three months, six months, adjust and get their patient ready for that. So, being able to advance the patient from point A to point B at the quickest pace possible . . . You need to be the director of the ship!"

But being "the director of the ship" was not easy for OPS therapists in the seas of physician authority in the hospital. OPS therapists had to negotiate this tension to validate their professional self, and this was evident in how they spoke about occupational norms. Nancy, a physical therapist, defined professionalism as "being self-disciplined, conducting yourself appropriately, and always wanting to help people—[being] someone who does the right thing for the patient, expressing concern and dedication to their patients . . . so that you don't harm them in any way." John, a speech therapist, reiterated this concern, saying, "You have the interests of the patient first, [such] that you will only treat a condition that you are trained to treat, [and] you wouldn't treat somebody if you didn't think they needed to be treated."

While physicians voiced concerns over "power trips" and "abuses of authority," OPS therapists spoke about occupational norms in terms of providing proper treatment for patients. The omission of any such abuses signaled their more modest position versus physicians, even when they viewed themselves as expert consultants. Furthermore, a majority of OPS therapists actually took ethics for granted, rarely discussing the topic or referring to it only in passing. Consequently, the moral individualism characteristic of physicians never surfaces in the professional self of OPS therapists, given their attenuated autonomy and control in the hospital.[15]

Although this suggests that it would be best to ignore the dissonance between being "director of the ship" and their subordinate role to physicians, OPS therapists found this hard to do, especially given the importance they placed on teamwork. All the OPS therapists felt that being a professional meant working well with others. Celia, an occupational therapist, explained that professionalism means "being able to collaborate with your colleagues, with the doctors, and [to] have a positive relation with them. . . . It's very important for us to be able to work with others so that [in] making competent recommendations we are respected . . . especially with physicians because that is what teamwork means for us."

While physicians embraced their role as the ultimate decision-makers and team leaders, OPS therapists insisted that teamwork involved being equal partners with physicians (though less often with other professionals, such as nurses). Yet equal respect and authority were scarce in Hospital General, and the OPS therapists seemed inclined to defend their status as partners on the team. Andrew's statement is representative:

> [A professional speech therapist is] somebody that works well with others, especially with the doctors . . . because we give them our recommendations and we can tell them, "This needs to be done and this is what is happening with this patient." A professional speech pathologist can work with . . . specialty physicians across the hospi-

tal . . . but there is so much we actually offer to physicians [because]
of our expertise and it's like we are both equal partners in the team.

Admitting to this occupational aspiration ("*it's like* we are both equal
partners in the team") intimates "equality without respect"—*together but
apart*—which may represent a defeat for OPS therapists who have constructed a professional self that is aligned with physicians while at the
same time safely distant from others below them. Here, in the relational
crux of teamwork, OPS therapists are found at their most dignified and
also most vulnerable.

The "Educated" Caregiver

Susie Smythe, a woman in her late forties and a registered nurse for fifteen
years, always talked about how often she felt like quitting. During her lunch
break one day, she confided why she felt that way: "It's always something
around here. Whether the doctors or other staff or the patients treat you
like you're there to serve them . . . or the administration who want us to do
more and more, we're in the middle, and we are the first ones to be blamed
for stuff." As I sympathized with her, she replied, "The thing is that we're
not seen as professionals. People have more respect for us now than they
did thirty years ago, but still, we have to fight for that all the time." Susie's
struggle framed how many nurses in Hospital General constructed a professional self.

Concerns over upgrading the status of nursing and disavowing degrading stereotypes are still relevant today.[16] Historically, nursing has
sought professional status primarily by standardizing nursing practice
and increasing educational requirements and credentials.[17] In Hospital
General, nurses were encouraged by their administrative colleagues to
participate in research, keep up with continuing education units, and obtain specialty credentials. Likewise, by providing financial support and
time off, the hospital encouraged nurses to pursue baccalaureate and
graduate-level degrees.

This historical context and workplace expectations serve as a backdrop for how nurses defined a professional in their field. Of all the groups
I interviewed, nurses were the most eager to discuss professionalism in
contrast to the enduring stereotypes of them as merely "bedpan-emptying

and butt-cleaning" attendants, "the bowel and bladder people," or "the doctor's handmaiden." Their discourse reflected a quest for recognition as they routinely confronted the humble origins of their occupation.[18] As Tanya lamented, "The poop and the puke and the deaf and the dying and the difficult families and the grunt work . . . [nursing is] very blue collar to some people . . . but there are registered nurses and there are bachelor degree nurses! I don't feel like I'm always changing diapers or always emptying puke. . . . Education kind of gives you a sense of pride and a way of saying 'We're professionals too!'"

Nurses struggled to construct a professional self in opposition to widely held views of nursing as unskilled work, and education promised to dispel these misconceptions. Overwhelmingly, the nurses I interviewed referred to formal education, obtaining credentials, or having a college degree as central to professionalism. In contrast to physicians and OPS therapists, who defined professionalism in terms of competently applying knowledge, nurses quite clearly wanted to have that knowledge in the first place. For James, the link between education and status for nurses was clear: "The more qualified you are and the more letters you have after your name, then the more money you can demand, the more respect and the more power you have . . . Also, it's about trying to get respect from the general public and others we work with: if we have a bachelors or master's degree then we can be seen as professionals."

Another nurse concurred: "A professional nurse is above all an educated nurse: she has to have formal education so that she is well informed, understands pharmacology, understands pathophysiology, understands the way people interact with one another. A professional nurse is a very good communicator and has excellent critical thinking skills, and that starts with having, as I said, formal education."

It was not, however, just any type of knowledge that nurses sought. Rather, they viewed formal education as a means to obtain the "right" knowledge— that of physicians' biomedical scientific approach to health care. But their emphasis on formal education was a catch-22, since a majority of nurses on the floor did not have more than a two-year associate's degree. The professional self was thus symbolically balanced on the shoulders of nurses who had made it to the top, "like Jenny Krause, who has a PhD and specializes in pediatric pain," as one nurse said enthusiastically.

This formulation is somewhat contrary to the concerns of Suzanne

Gordon and Sioban Nelson, who argue, in *The Complexities of Care: Nursing Reconsidered*, that nurses utilize a discourse of caring that neglects their biomedical skills in favor of a mythical Nightingale image of "soft skills."[19] Though I heard this discourse frequently, I also noticed efforts to redefine the caring nurses perform in ways that validated their knowledge and skills. As one nurse reflected, the skills associated with caring were routinely dismissed, as if the tacit skills borne of experience tacked well behind those acquired in the classroom:

> Okay, this is the one thing [about caring work] that blows my
> mind. . . . At the core of nursing is caring that goes beyond the
> body, beyond the biological and physiological. It's something that
> most people don't know how to do, and [that] you can't always
> measure, and this has been used to the detriment of nurses because
> this work is not necessarily seen as professional work or as knowl-
> edgeable work, and as us having real skills . . . like doctors. . . . Car-
> ing is the number one thing we [nurses] have: you can give people
> medicines up the wazoo but . . . sitting down and knowing how to
> talk with the patient and working with them [patients] takes a lot
> [of] skills to get them to where they need to be. . . . We know how
> and when to do this.

Though a majority of the nurses I spoke with emphasized their command of biomedical knowledge in patient health and well-being, they frequently did so in the context of *wanting* more formal education rather than *having* such knowledge and skills by virtue of their experience with patients.[20]

While rejecting the prevailing image of nurses as unskilled workers, they also emphasized occupational norms in constructing a professional self. "A professional nurse has ethics," Patti explained. They are "someone who's honest, caring, definitely confidential, making the patients and their families feel . . . like he's their only patient and that they want the best for that patient." For nurses, ethics meant something different than it did for physicians or even OPS therapists—ethics was not about "power tripping" or "do no harm." Instead, as described by Joe, a professional nurse must be willing to "put [themselves] aside for the job. You put yourself aside for the patient." Joe, a nurse in an intensive care unit, further explained that professionalism is "not to neglect yourself, but sometimes you have to do that." But in emphasizing their selfless commitment to others beyond their own needs, the nurses' professional self was conflicted in relation to their quest for formal education and occupational mobility (i.e., pay and status). In this context, the yearning for professional control and autonomy may contradict widely held traditional images of nursing.[21]

Nurses negotiated this tension by integrating teamwork as the third dimension of their professional self. They explained that professionalism meant fulfilling a mediating and coordinating role on the health-care team. "Nurses make sure everybody is on the same page," one nurse told me. As Kathy put it, a nurse is someone who "tries to make it all work and makes sure that everybody is working together. You [as a professional nurse] are there to teach others like residents, [and to] teach patients and their families. . . . It's about teamwork and trying to put all the parts of the puzzle together."

Clearly, nurses "oiled the machinery," viewing themselves as "brokers" on the health-care team, which is not surprising given how often they felt caught in the middle of the hospital's occupational hierarchy. While her conclusions are debatable, Davina Allen has argued that the nurses' role as coordinators may be their best occupational strategy for upgrading their tenuous status.[22] Yet they seemed to rescue some dignity by highlighting how their position allowed them to "teach" others—practitioners and patients/families alike. Their professional self was able to integrate its desire to be seen as an "educated" practitioner by diligently invoking a caring ethics.[23] Professional nurses gave of themselves—and their knowledge and expertise (however defined)—to others. Using an interesting analogy, Ruby elaborated: "It's not just being knowledgeable, having the education . . . It's kind of like you are teaching the patient a dance. Patients come to this institution, and they are totally blown away by how crazy it is in here [in the hospital]. . . . And you [as a professional nurse] have to do that [teach them the dance] with [a] certain finesse." Here, the dance instructor merges with the choreographer, lending nurses a degree of symbolic importance, which they are routinely denied in Hospital General. This professional self embodies sensitivity and sensibility, and in the context of their limited autonomy and power, both in the hospital and historically, nurses make the best of their role and what they claim as their own specialty—educated caring.[24]

The Skeptical Technician

It was not uncommon to hear respiratory therapists debate occupational issues, but on one occasion a heated conversation that had ensued over "changes" in the department abruptly ended when the new department manager walked in. As I walked with Roy toward the ICU, he revisited the topic. "Well, since we have this manager, there's been a push to be more professional," he said sarcastically, "but that is BS. . . . We do our jobs, deal with the respiratory stuff, and that's it." When I asked what he thought the manager meant by being "more professional," Roy explained that "she's talking about more training and education," and about the therapists acting and conducting themselves "with respect, as experts in respiratory issues." But for Roy, even a graduate degree wouldn't elevate the status of respiratory therapists, "'cause we just don't have the authority that docs have." Hearing Roy's disenchantment, I wondered if he almost resents the notion of being a professional.

Emerging after World War II as an offspring of pulmonary medicine, respiratory therapy is a young occupation that assumed some of the bedside tasks previously performed by nurses. Recently, it has struggled to transcend its publicly devalued technical status by bringing attention to its advanced and specialized proficiency in respiratory interventions. Still, fragmented efforts to raise the occupational status of respiratory therapy through educational credentials have proven futile. Respiratory therapy remains one of the many technical occupations in the hospital that have no autonomy from physicians' supervision and direction.[25] The therapists' inability to surpass the limits of their role provides the background for how they view their job and their relationship to other practitioners on the floor.[26]

In this context, respiratory therapists (RTs) constructed a professional self narrowly, defining it as having knowledge of the technology. This was typically followed by a disclaimer that more formal education was "unnecessary" because it was no guarantee of more status in the hospital. "It [a bachelor's degree] is useless for what our work involves, really," Annie sighed, in a resigned tone. For RTs, it was difficult to imagine the professional self apart from purely technical tasks, but they tried. "We are very technical people, like x-ray techs. . . . We are very, very good at technology," Jon explained. "It's amazing what we [RTs] can manage in terms of technology." During interviews, sullen resignation often turned into exaltation, especially when RTs discussed their role with patients. As Tom, a senior RT in the ICU, enthusiastically explained: "Do you realize what I mean when I say to ventilate someone? It takes a certain pressure to get air into someone's lungs and there are adjustments that we can make on our very, very complicated microprocessing equipment that runs as a ventilator. There are adjustments that we make so that pressure is not too high. . . . Those fine-tuning things can really save a patient's life!"

While RTs resisted a professional self centered on credentials, they tried to cash in on the only "ticket to fame" they believed they had. Through working with complex machines and having knowledge of respiratory technology—or, as one RT put it, "knowing how to manage equipment"—one could hear the faint echo of a professional self.

In this light, very few RTs viewed professionalism in terms of occupational norms. As Tammy put it, professionalism "is a loaded issue. First and foremost, professionalism is doing the right thing; you've got to be a patient advocate, considering the patient's family or the patients. . . . You have to be able to behave with all those people in an appropriate way. So I guess it is about having the ethical values, knowing how to behave, and having the patient's interests in the forefront."

The issue was not that RTs conceived of occupational norms differently from other practitioners, but that very few of them actually talked about this dimension even when probed. This was understandable, for they had no authority to grapple with the norms, nor could they determine treatment for a patient; they generally followed orders even when, as we will see, they had good reasons not to.

Talking about teamwork did not offer respiratory therapists much respite either, even though a majority of them identified it as a dimension of professionalism. Typically, teamwork meant effectively communicating some degree of their knowledge of technology to other practitioners. As Roxy explained, "We have to establish good relationships with other staff and we have to present ourselves in a pleasant and professional manner by communicating well with everybody. . . . We have to be able to explain to others what this ventilator is doing, why the setting is this and not that, etc."

The professional self of the RTs was tenuous, resting on what the status hierarchy relegated to the shallow soil of technical expertise. In essence, the RTs' contribution to teamwork was translating: helping other practitioners (and, on occasion, patients/families) make sense of what they do technically.

The Emotional Supporter

The social services department was always welcoming, and the social workers frequently spoke of how social work "fit" in the hospital. They were all quite candid about the challenges their department faced and about feeling marginal in the hospital environment—particularly Lori, a woman in her mid-forties with over seventeen years in the field. "What happens is that we always come last," she said, shaking her head in disappointment. "We don't do the medical things and they see us as expendable. They think we're only here for the welfare paper sort of thing, paperwork, [to] do secretary stuff . . . but we are licensed, with a master's degree." Social workers commonly felt dismissed and devalued when they spoke of their peripheral role in Hospital General.

The history of social work is characterized, perhaps as much as nursing, by efforts to achieve professional standing via medicine's model, especially in relation to psychiatry.[27] But social work has struggled as its claims to expertise have been contested and because the clinical and reform branches of the occupation are divided, with the former pursuing a professional model similar to that of physicians, and the latter focusing politically on community activism and social change.[28] By the early 1900s, medical social work emerged as a specialization by adopting scientific principles and standards. Medicine as an institution has influenced social workers' practice, especially in the hospital, where physicians frequently decide when social work is necessary. On the other hand, like OPS therapists, social workers are licensed to practice autonomously in providing services such as individual or family psychological counseling.

In Hospital General, this larger context framed the social workers' views of professionalism. They defined professionalism in terms of their "clinical expertise," highlighting their knowledge of brain functioning, psychology, and therapeutic skills. But they found it difficult to represent themselves in ways that were meaningful to other practitioners. As one social worker put it, "It's not easy to explain in this environment what we do and why we are professionals too . . . especially because we [social workers] have a different type of knowledge. It is definitely different from the medical knowledge everybody else has in the hospital."

Social workers struggled to find common ground with other practitioners as an essential part of the health-care world they shared, often leaving the professional self exposed and lacking validation. Though finding validation was a constant challenge, it was not impossible. Robert described being a professional as "having clinical confidence" and using one's clinical skills and knowledge base. He emphasized that there was more to social work than just specialized training:

> [There are] psychiatrists that have distinguished degrees from elite universities and a pile of really high-quality knowledge but they do not have the personality to be a therapist, to be a clinician. They don't have the heart, the ability to empathize, the ability to step outside oneself and see emotion and pain and the reality of somebody else's life and develop clinical knowledge and skills like us. [A professional is] someone who has the principles of the heart and the training.

For social workers, the professional self was an expert of the "heart," and this was based not on something that could be standardized and practiced uniformly (such as biomedical or technical knowledge) but on the intangible quality of one's personality. Professionalism entailed cultivating the "right" personal temperament in relating to others (usually in suffering). Social workers saw their expertise in terms of personal virtues that were enhanced through formal training and work experience to better integrate the emotional, social, and physical aspects of health care. Unfortunately, this professional self was always on the defensive, as social workers were viewed as "nonmedical folk" regardless of how much specialized knowledge or how many clinical skills they had accumulated.

Social workers also considered occupational norms a critical aspect of the professional self.[29] But, they interpreted these differently, going beyond the typical statements from other groups (such as "having integrity," "behaving appropriately," and "being honest"). As Judith explained, "I think you have to be aware of how you feel about certain things. Like, if you're working with someone who maybe is in jail for a horrible crime, you have to ask yourself, 'Can I work with this person? Can I be nonjudgmental and care for this person?' I think people would get in over their heads if they tried to do something they are not necessarily prepared for at this level."

When discussing professional ethics, social workers showcased all the symbolic effort they had invested in becoming "experts of the heart." As Dave explained, ethical conduct required "knowing where to draw the line":

> [A professional social worker is] someone who can give of them-
> selves without giving away themselves—someone who maintains
> professional ethical boundaries, [so] that you can be involved but
> not over-involved. . . . Someone who has the ability to be with a
> patient, no matter how painful that can be, but do it in the appropri-
> ate way, not losing themselves in the process. . . . Again, boundaries
> I think are a very big thing for us in terms of professionalism.

What is interesting here is how social workers understood their emotional involvement in ethical terms: knowing how and when to restrain their emotions was central to conducting themselves appropriately. If one recalls how physicians discussed occupational norms, they too spoke of the ethics of restraining their emotions and not giving in to power trips. Yet for social workers, setting emotional and relationship boundaries was a catch-22, as it undermined their efforts to legitimate a professional self in an organizational context of biomedical science; it reinforced how different social workers were from the valued currency of biomedical expertise in the hospital. Autonomy on the margins was bittersweet indeed.

An overwhelming majority of the social workers I interviewed regarded teamwork as an important element of professionalism, even though it offered an unsatisfying resolution to their marginality. According to Tess, "social workers have the ability to relate to other professionals" and to "develop really core relationships with them" so that everyone on a team "can rely on each other's assessments and feel confident that each side has done their job." Put another way, social workers contribute to their teams by "giving assistance to all the parties involved in the process." Social workers viewed themselves as the emotional supporters of the team, "lending a hand" by assisting with and building relationships among its members. Another social worker elaborated on this role:

[A professional social worker] provides assistance to the medical team. You have nurses that are at the bedside of a child and they're completely breaking down. Sometimes, after you've helped the family, you have to take that time to listen to them [other practitioners]. I don't think they [other practitioners] realize that, but sometimes we're their support system as well, to keep them going, to do what they have to do. We're really part of the team to help them as much as patients. It's about assisting others in whatever capacity . . . But building a relationship with that nurse or that physician takes work!

But even when social workers found a concrete role, such as the team's therapist, this hardly conferred much status among a cadre of other practitioners performing "life-saving" work; a professional self forged on being the emotional supporter failed to deliver validation. In some ways, social workers found themselves in a more vulnerable position than RTs, whose knowledge of technology ultimately provided them with a common language in relating to other groups, such as physicians and nurses. What emerges in the social workers' efforts to validate their professional status is how emotions—as a knowledge area and the object of work—represent an asset and a liability. Even though health-care work requires incredible levels of emotional labor, the hospital does not nurture what practitioners must summon from within. Addressing this void, social workers stood faithful and dignified in recognition of their undervalued yet critical position in the expert—biomedical—world of Hospital General.[30]

Professionalism Reconsidered

The world of the professional is different from the world of most workers—it commands respect, and it is dignified labor. This is even truer of the working lives of health-care practitioners in Hospital General, a setting of almost sacred dimensions, where life and death frequently hang in the balance. But, for the women and men I interviewed (with the notable exception of the physicians), respect was elusive, and dignity a fragile state. Upon discussing the professional self, a topic that most people take for granted, it became clearer just how hard it was for health-care practitioners to attain the secure and certain identity that so much of the literature on professionalism portrays. The hierarchical division of health-care labor was an ever-present reminder that not all professionals are created equal, nor is the distribution of symbolic (and material) rewards.

Though different professional selves emerge from the occupational histories and work experiences of the practitioners introduced in this chapter, professionalism is still hegemonic in the hospital insofar as it incorporates variation without abdicating its exclusionary nature. Apart from *what* they said, the voices and the demeanor of the practitioners conveyed membership in a prestigious endeavor (though with reservations among the RTs). This, however, was a distinction from the world of most human labor that barely mattered when considered in relation to other health-care workers, where different occupational concerns corresponded to the prestige of each groups' knowledge base.[31]

The social organization of hospital work also brought an interesting new dimension to professionalism—teamwork and team membership. Teamwork constitutes a relatively less explored dimension of the professional self compared to knowledge and normative behaviors. Unlike physicians, who tried to ennoble their role as the ultimate medical authorities (at least formally), all the other groups sought to integrate teamwork in ways that did not betray the essential nature of the professional self—that of the autonomy to control one's labor, based on the deployment of esoteric knowledge. Ideas about teamwork brought to light the uneasy relationship between the groups' desires to be seen as professionals and the reality of how teams operate—who does what, who answers to who, who gets to say what is to be done. The ideological work of practitioners trying to make teamwork a meaningful dimension of the professional self reflected occupational struggles within the organization of health care in the hospital, and the jury is still out on the promise of an authentic partnership. Teamwork has become emblematic of health care in general, and it was certainly highlighted in the organizational culture of Hospital General, as we shall see in the following chapter. But it did not adequately address the existing tensions and inconsistencies in how the groups related to one another and how they viewed the others' roles. The professional self is most malleable, least certain, and *most at risk* when practitioners must work side by side and occupational boundaries become blurred or are crossed. Hospital work forces practitioners to confront each other's larger occupational baggage; they see in each other not only what they do not want to become but also what they all want to achieve or protect. In short, professional selves are reproduced in tension with others, yet they cannot succeed without each other.

One issue that remains when considering the professional self is where and how caring fits into the picture. It was rather surprising, for example, that while mostly nurses and social workers hinted at caring, it was not a significant aspect of how they conceived of professionalism. This raises the question of whether professionalism can provide the space for caring if knowledge (of a certain kind) remains its preeminent pursuit. I believe a key reason that caring is absent from practitioner conceptions of professionalism is because it has been subsumed within the teamwork ideal; that is, under teamwork, no one occupation is singled out to provide caring, because it is "the team" that cares for patients. By abstracting care into this symbolic space, the teamwork ideal obscures not only the occupational hierarchy but also who is responsible for caring (i.e., "if everyone is here to care, maybe someone else will cover my back for now").[32] But before I address the issue of caring more fully, I will turn to how practitioners interact with each other on the floor. As is often said, "What people say is one thing, and what they do is another," and as I conducted my research, I wondered how the professional self maintained its integrity in light of its most vulnerable dimension—the teamwork culture of the hospital.

Chapter 2

Teamwork in the Hospital

I think we all try hard to walk the talk, as they say.
—OCCUPATIONAL THERAPIST

HEALTH TEAM NEWS, the hospital's newsletter, had announced the staff appreciation lunch, an annual tradition. Plans had been made on the floor about who would take time off to attend and bring lunch back for those staying behind. On the day of the lunch, I walked with the staff toward the center of the hospital campus, where large white tents, umbrellas, and round tables with chairs filled a big parking lot, blocking off two internal streets. There were stands selling discounted pain relievers and offering many free goodies, as well as information booths. There was live music and raffle prizes, and upwards of one thousand staff lined up for the abundant food.

After a few hours, the event organizer, the vice chair of the staff assembly executive committee, thanked everyone for their hard work. "We appreciate each other—the diversity of everyone here," she said enthusiastically. "This is why we are a great institution. . . . We have so many wonderful teams providing the best care for our patients." People applauded as they ate lunch. The event exuded high morale, camaraderie, and esprit de corps; I found myself feeling proud of being part of the moment.

Inside the hospital, hall posters and pamphlets promoted a well-coordinated, harmonious "health care team" composed of highly trained, caring practitioners involved not just in patient care but also in health research. Hospital General's website also advertised this depiction of its staff.

40

Conversation on the floor referred to those providing care as "the team," highlighting the organizational culture of the hospital and its public image. This was not just any team—it was a team of *professionals* whose collective efforts served the health-care needs of patients and their families. It was surprising how much emphasis was placed daily on this idea of an "expert health care team at your service" (as one of the pamphlets read). Why was so much effort dedicated to something that is almost assumed to be a given in today's health-care delivery? Perhaps there was more than met the eye to this idea of teamwork among professionals.

The teamwork concept has generally been studied in blue-collar industrial settings, especially during the 1970s and 1980s, when rank-and-file industrial workers were called on to collaborate not only with each other, on participatory work teams, but also with management, to improve the production process and company performance.[1] Applied to professional work settings, the idea of teamwork at first glance appears redundant, given that by definition professionals are expected to work collaboratively—even democratically—in providing services. Yet this understanding is based on considering a single professional occupation, be it attorneys, accountants, or university faculty—*not* in considering different professional groups working collectively in the same setting, for outside the hospital context this seldom happens.

Because the term "team" does not specify or identify any formalized grouping of practitioners with explicit roles and codified rights and responsibilities, I view the rhetoric of "teams" and "teamwork" as obscuring the occupational hierarchy and who has the authority to decide on diagnosis and treatment.[2] Not only must each group confront the organizational constraints of the hospital, they also have to square off against each other in what Andrew Abbott termed "jurisdictional disputes," which challenge professional autonomy based on claims to expert knowledge.[3] In this sense, each group is part of the health-care team, but because the knowledge claims of each group are ranked hierarchically, the collaborative nature of teamwork is tenuous, and the results frequently a dissonant clash of roles rather than the symphonic harmony upheld and promoted by the hospital administration. Why else would the hospital invest such significant symbolic and material resources to celebrate this ideal of teamwork?

The tension between the hospital culture of teamwork and practitioner conceptions of professionalism became apparent during the research I discussed in the previous chapter, where I interviewed groups struggling to integrate teamwork as a key element of their professional selves. In referring to a hospital culture, I am focusing on administrative efforts to promote certain ideals and images that define the hospital not only for the public but also in the hearts and minds of staff and practitioners. The annual staff appreciation lunch exemplifies a ritualistic gathering where such symbolism is reinforced, as it is in the public displays of teamwork throughout the hospital corridors and in media advertising throughout the region. Workshops and conferences sponsored by the hospital and attended by employed staff, visiting practitioners, and the public also promote what one might consider "preferred readings" of Hospital General, which tend to—*or are intended to*—put forward its best face or flatter it. This formal hospital culture may be contrasted with the informal hospital culture of understandings shared by those working there; that is, the folklore, inside jokes, atrocity stories, water cooler talk, gossip, and scuttlebutt, as well as the norms that operate beneath the purview of the public (though not always that of the patients).

So while practitioners may verbally embrace the teamwork ideal, the ethnographic evidence suggests that it is neither easy to be part of the team nor to have a legitimate voice on it—even when one is considered to have expert skills. The cracks in the teamwork ideal become evident through three sets of behaviors on the floor: (1) paying lip service to teamwork, which was done primarily by physicians, (2) finding a legitimate voice on the team, which was most evident among OPS therapists, and social workers, and less so among nurses, and (3) practicing solo, which was the case for RTs and nurses to some extent. In the end, teamwork was less an organizational ideal in Hospital General and more an *ideology* in a field of struggle. Rachael Finn and her colleagues have argued that "the system of professions, with a historically developed, institutionalized set of hierarchical relations between them . . . supports fundamentally different professional interests. Consequently, we suggest the tendency is likely to be towards conflict and contestation, to the detriment of team integration."[4] As the following scenes illustrate, collaboration is not something that can be guaranteed, but rather something that must be worked at as practitioners labor to project their professional status in the context of an organizational hierarchy of expertise.[5]

We All Belong: Lip Service to Teamwork

In the vernacular of hospital staff, the ICUs are "a totally different world," and the people working in them are "creatures of a different kind." One morning, while I was getting acquainted with the nurses and other staff in one of the ICUs, an attending physician entered the unit. As fellows, residents, nurses, and a respiratory therapist joined him just outside one of the glass-enclosed rooms, the activity in the rest of the unit slowed down.

After reviewing the patient's chart, the attending asked a senior resident about the results of some tests. The resident, who had just awakened from a nap, was obviously drowsy but unfazed; turning to a young woman wearing an impeccable white coat, the resident asked her to "present" on the patient. The woman, a second-year resident, frantically recited the patient's history, lab results, current treatment, potential future complications, and possible treatments.

Everyone was quiet, and after a few seconds the attending authoritatively asked her why she had diagnosed this patient as she did. The junior resident stammered out an answer that clearly did not satisfy the attending physician. No one came to her rescue, and two young male residents could barely contain their smirks. The situation was awkward and the tension was growing.

"Dr. Grant, I do not wish to make you uncomfortable," the attending said sternly, "but it is part of being a competent professional to be able to consider alternative diagnoses, and my questioning is only directed at making you a better physician. Have you asked nursing, who by the way is part of our team, what their thoughts are on the abnormal levels of creatinine?"

The resident, embarrassed, murmured an almost imperceptible "I understand" as the attending turned to a nurse for his opinion. Peter, an RN, provided an elaborate explanation on kidney function, followed by a detailed history of the patient he had cared for intermittently over the past year. He then described specific physical manifestations of the kidney problem that had been detected by the blood work.

Satisfied with Peter's assessment, the attending physician turned to Dr. Grant to make sure she had been paying attention. He then asked Tim, the RT, if there was anything he would like to add. After Tim briefly explained the patient's respiratory status, the attending asked for other opinions before explaining why the patient had presented abnormal lab results and what the appropriate course of treatment should be. The other residents were taking notes and nodding in approval.

Dr. Grant, the junior resident, was still trying to recover her composure as people shuffled to the patient next door. "We are part of a medical team," the attending reiterated to the group. "We are here as physicians working with nurses and other staff who are professionals in their own areas. . . . I hope you have all realized that today, because you should be asking them about their assessments. . . . We work with each other." This was certainly true, though what was obscured *and reproduced* through this incident— one repeated frequently at Hospital General—was the ranking of expertise and status hierarchy among occupational groups, in which physicians directed the team and ultimately had the final say.

Upon entering Labor and Delivery (L&D), I was embraced by a silence so peaceful that I feared my squeaking shoes would disturb this sanctuary. I spent the morning with Gayle, one of the L&D nurses, who had worked in this unit since becoming a registered nurse many years ago. "You are just in time for the action," she said, as her patient was about to give birth. Having never witnessed a delivery, I smiled in nervous anticipation of whatever awaited me behind the patient's door. Gayle was in full charge of her domain as she handled equipment, administered drugs, and kept up with tedious charting. The patient and her husband followed Gayle's instructions as she calmly explained everything she was doing and what would be happening sequentially until the baby was born.

As the attending physician and residents arrived, Gayle respectfully deferred to them and, using technical vocabulary, described the status of the patient and the baby to the physicians. The residents listened closely as the attending responded to Gayle in an equally technical manner, as if they were employing a secret language understood only by "the chosen." The residents politely asked the patient some health-related questions while one of them performed a "quick check" of her cervix, confirming its degree of dilation to evaluate the progression of labor. After the attending said that everything was going as expected, the doctors left, indicating that they would return later. Gayle turned back to the patient and her husband, who then bombarded her with questions about what the doctors had told Gayle (they had "not understood a word"). As she translated what the attending physician had said, Gayle simplified her language so that we all could understand the content and significance of his assessment.

After the new residents delivered the baby with no complications, their relief was palpable: they believed they had performed the most amazing of tricks. But it was Gayle who had done the hard work, constantly mediating and coordinating between patient, physicians, respiratory therapist, and other staff. She was able to accomplish this not only because of her extensive experience, but also because she had the "right" knowledge, something that garnered her much respect among her peers and other practitioners.

Things seemed to slow down after the delivery, and the attending, the residents, other nurses, Gayle, and I all mingled around the nurses' station. The attending told me I was lucky to be following Gayle since "she is so knowledgeable." As I nodded, smiling, the physician turned to Gayle: "Aren't you, Gayle, going for your master's?"

"Yes," Gayle answered.

The physician concluded, "That is why she is so great—she's continuing her education. . . . Gayle, you could still become a doctor . . . but you know that takes so many years in school . . . It's so much more difficult, all the stuff you have to learn in med school." Gayle graciously accepted the backhanded compliment, but her smile was bittersweet: while the physician may have not intended to demean her, the conversation exemplified how knowledgeable nurses such as Gayle are nevertheless subtly reminded of their subordinate status.

During a short break, Gayle shared with me some interesting stories about her experiences on the floor. Through the years, she had learned "how important it is to work as a team with doctors, residents and other staff." I asked about her role on that team and she passionately expressed how essential nurses are for the hospital, the patients, and "even for the rest of the staff." She explained that nurses "are constantly mediating and arranging things so that everything goes well for everybody." As she finished articulating her thoughts, her beeper sounded and we headed back to the patient's room.

Ideally, teamwork integrates expertise through intergroup collaboration on the floor. This was frequently evident in focused teaching rounds and in-services, where practitioners provided feedback and talked with each other in formalized ways. But the "expert health care team" was not a team of equals. Important disparities existed among practitioners, and as shown in the first vignette in this section, physician authority still held sway. This is perhaps why everyone (including physicians, to a degree) struggled to articulate teamwork as part of a professional self that was not contradicted by work experiences on the floor.

The ICU vignette also illustrates how the structure of hospital work privileged those with biomedical diagnostic skills—that is, primarily physicians, though others (such as nurses) frequently displayed diagnostic knowledge and routinely deployed it. The more I observed practitioners collaborating, the more I was struck by how routinely the teamwork ideal faltered when physicians permitted and validated input from other groups. In short, the team of experts resembled professionals ordering other professionals around, in terms of what, how, and when to do something. Consequently, I came to see how a teamwork ideology eased collective social-psychological tensions that were rooted in the hierarchical structure of expertise. Teamwork provided a framework for how to *feel* rather than to *think* about work, assuaging the collective anxiety—and perhaps also the resentment—that could easily emerge (and often did!) from such unequal relationships on the floor.

Wanting to Belong: Finding a Legitimate Voice on the Team

As I made my way through a busy corridor in the oldest wing of Hospital General, I smelled the odor of disinfectant and heard the animated voices of people in the background. When I arrived at the physical medicine and rehabilitation unit, which served patients undergoing acute physical rehabilitation, as well as neurology patients (i.e., individuals recovering from stroke, head injuries, or brain surgery), I was surprised by how terribly busy this unit seemed, how crowded everything was, and how indifferent the staff was to my presence. This unit is where OPS therapists help a variety of patients with rehabilitation, and I was in the way.

After finding a place where I could stand without being trampled, I heard one of the nurses calling for a speech therapist. A resident physician, Dr. Peterson, wanted a newly admitted stroke patient evaluated for swallowing. I followed the nurse as she juggled her papers, got medications from a drug-dispensing machine, and headed to the patient's room. She checked the patient and administered intravenous medication as Dr. Peterson explained what he wanted for the patient, including the consult from speech therapy she'd requested for him. The patient lay in bed, immobile, covered by white linen up to his waist. His eyes were closed and his hands rested on each side of his body.

Throughout the day, I saw physical and occupational therapists help patients move about their rooms, teaching them how to get out of bed or to carefully take a step. The patience and the dedication of the therapists was astonishing, as it took each patient a long time to complete motions such as stepping forward half a foot or slowly and awkwardly curling their stiff fingers around a large plastic cup; at times, there was no progress at all.

As I greeted Celia, one of the speech therapists, Dr. Peterson approached her on behalf of the newly admitted patient. "Would you mind assessing him?" he asked. He did not believe that the patient had a swallowing deficiency "since the stroke was very mild and we caught it in time, but I need you to tell me what really is going on."

Celia carefully examined the patient by opening his mouth, feeling around his jaw, and asking him "yes or no" questions, which the patient answered with nods and headshakes. Celia continued her assessment by giving the patient a thick nectar-like fluid, which he was able to suck with a straw and swallow without any problems.

One hour and many tests later, we headed to the nurses' station, where Celia wrote her evaluation and paged Dr. Peterson. When he called back, Celia explained the patient's health status, made her recommendation regarding his diet and head-rest position, and suggested some further specialized testing to fully rule out any other problems, given the patient's stroke diagnosis. The physician agreed to follow Celia's recommendation only after a lengthy conversation, during which he seemed to want the last word about the treatment and prognosis of "his" patient.

During a follow-up interview, Celia told me about a similar conversation with another physician, one who "just had a mindset" about his patient's condition and accused the nurses of paranoia for insisting that the patient was having trouble with swallowing. This physician told Celia to recheck the patient, saying that "I think he is really fine, and these people [the nurses] are wrong." After quizzing the doctor about the patient's injuries, however, Celia concluded that the patient was definitely a candidate for dysphagia (difficulty swallowing). After she saw the patient, she stated that she "would recommend nothing per mouth"; moreover, she felt he needed to have a swallowing x-ray and to be seen by an ENT [ears, nose, and throat] specialist. The resident reacted to Celia's recommendation by being gruff and confrontational, but the ENT doctors confirmed what she suspected: the patient had a paralyzed vocal cord.

"It took so much energy to settle the issue," Celia said. Her conversations with the residents illustrate a struggle for respect that was present in numerous therapist-physician interactions.

The pediatric unit is spacious, well lighted, and colorfully decorated. The children's themes on the walls make the unit less frightening for children and parents alike. Russ, a social worker, asked how my project was going, and I asked if I might shadow him during his rounds. As I had anticipated, Russ hesitated a bit and explained that there were many privacy issues with the patients he dealt with. It would be fine, however, if I observed his visit with Kelly, since he would not be doing "therapy per se" in her case. Thus, I stood quietly in a corner of Kelly's room as I watched Russ provide emotional and psychological support to the patient and her family.

Kelly was a fifteen-year-old who had been diagnosed with advanced bone cancer and had been recently transferred to the floor from the ICU. As the nurse checked the IV bag and the pump next to the young girl, Russ stood close by and listened intently to Kelly's mother as she spoke, her voice cracking. Russ reassured the clearly distressed woman that the physicians would do everything possible to give Kelly the best treatment. As a gesture of support, he placed his hand on the mother's shoulder, resting it there momentarily; it conveyed heartfelt sympathy without being overly sentimental or expressing dismay or pity.

How could Russ do this work day in and day out for so many years? His voice was steady and calm as he responded to the family's questions and eased the doubts of a frightened young girl. Meanwhile, the pediatric oncologist, who had entered the room with me, remained unmoved and unaltered—simply an observer in the background, just like me—while the nurse sat on the bed, holding Kelly's hand.

Russ eventually turned to the physician and suggested that Kelly might need some time to think about the treatment options with her parents. "OK, you can let me know when you have made your decision," the physician replied. "I will be around later." Russ spoke with the family again, gave them his card, and assured them that he would be available whenever they needed him. They thanked him profusely for his support.

Later, as I sat at the nurses' station, I listened to an intense discussion between Russ and the oncologist. The physician seemed upset because the parents had not decided to proceed with his recommended treatment and because they wanted to consider other opinions. Russ stood his ground, firmly stating that the oncologist could not be "putting pressure on them like that to make a decision" and that Russ's job as "a professional was to make sure their rights were respected." While Russ could not evaluate the medical treatment, he told the physician that the family needed more time and he would assist them emotionally for what they were about to face.

Visibly annoyed, the physician curtly ended the conversation with "OK, let me know when they've made a decision." By the time Russ finished his paperwork, the day shift was ending and the family had yet to make a decision.

Once again, the "expert health-care team" sounds better in theory than in reality. Practitioners routinely had to defend their role on the team and remind others of their expertise and the legitimacy of their opinion in treating patients. As the speech therapist's vignette highlight, claiming a collaborative role required that practitioners effectively challenge the knowledge and authority of physicians. That practitioners such as speech therapists and social workers searched for a (*respected*) voice was another indication that the teamwork ideal was difficult to uphold in the course of patient care. These confrontations, especially as the social worker's vignette illustrates, testify to the tension between the leveling character of the teamwork ideology and the organizational status hierarchy. Physicians felt they could override the roles of other practitioners, but other practitioners seldom returned the insult.

Ironically, the social worker and speech therapist vignettes may actually represent an attempt to fulfill the promise of teamwork on the floor. Unlike nurses and respiratory therapists, OPS therapists and social workers can practice independently outside the hospital without physician supervision. Because of this, they were more likely than nurses and RTs to assert themselves and resort not only to their knowledge base but also to ethics arguments when they felt undermined by inauthentic collaboration in treating patients. Of all the groups, OPS therapists and social workers had more opportunity to resist physician dominance, validate their expertise, and dignify both their professional self and the romanticized version of team-work endorsed by the hospital. A further irony is that, particularly among OPS therapists, this quest for a respected voice on the team often meant that they exercised authority over others, such as nurses, and thus they reproduced much of the hierarchical, contested relations that they experi-enced and resisted themselves.

Practicing Solo: Working Alone on the Team

I arrived at the Respiratory Department as Teresa, the night supervisor, was preparing paperwork and making sure the other RTs had their assign-ments and patient reports. She told me I would follow Dan during the early evening, the "most exciting" time. Then, as patients fell asleep and things slowed down, I could spend the rest of the shift with her, since she was in charge of patients in the emergency room, and as everyone knows, "there's always something going on there." Having been an RT in Hospital General for almost three decades, Dan was no stranger to the night shift. He wel-comed me and asked if I was ready to "hit the floor." As we walked through the long, lonely, and quiet corridors, he detailed his routine in an authorita-tive tone.

After arriving at one of the ICUs, which was where all of his patients were located, he looked at his notes and decided to start with the "old guy." As we made our way toward this patient's room, a nurse approached and asked Dan to check her patient's ventilator settings since "they don't seem right to me." Dan asked whether it was urgent, to which the nurse replied that the patient's oxygen was a little bit low and his color was different. Dan hesitated momentarily, as if he needed a bit more information to decide on whether to check this one patient. The nurse advised us to gown up because the patient was in isolation. When I asked why he was isolated, the nurse and Dan both looked at me and then replied in unison with an acronym I had never heard of.

As we headed to the patient's room, I was unsure about whether I wanted to follow Dan inside. Dan noticed my uneasiness and assured me that I would be able to see and hear everything if I stood just outside the large sliding glass door of the small ICU room.

Dan put on his isolation gown, gloves, and mask, and walked toward the ventilator at the bedside. He glanced at a wide chart that the RTs used to keep track of a patient's status, respiratory assessments, treatments, medications, and ventilator settings. He then quickly looked at the patient and focused his attention on the ventilator. As he pressed buttons on the machine, it beeped, and digital numbers traversed its small screen. After quite a while, he looked at me and said, enthusiastically, "I figured it out—one of the settings was not right for him." Dan then turned to the patient (who seemed to be sleeping but was actually unconscious) and made sure that the tube entering his throat was properly positioned. He lightly adjusted the mechanical arm holding the plastic tube through which air flowed from the ventilator into the patient's lungs. Appearing satisfied, he jotted down something on the chart and walked back to me while removing his disposable gloves and gown.

As I followed him around the unit from room to room, his routine became somewhat predictable, even to my untrained eye. He would approach a ventilator, read the chart, fiddle with the machine, make some adjustments to the positioning of the equipment, chart the changes he made, and leave the room. Dan interacted more with the equipment than with either the patients or the other practitioners with whom he might confer.

Teamwork proved a lonelier experience for some practitioners than others, and practicing solo on the hospital's expert team meant being either at the top or at the bottom. For those at the top—primarily physicians—working solo resonated with the moral individualism of their professional self. But for others, such as respiratory therapists, practicing solo rendered their work less significant.[6] More than for any other group, the work of RTs revealed a gnawing schism between the teamwork ideal and their professional self, as the performance of their machines seemed to overshadow any knowledge they had acquired through formal training or workplace experience. This put the specter of deskilling front-and-center for RTs—a fear commonly associated with industrial manual labor rather than professionalized occupations.[7] This is not to say that other groups did not face similar threats to the professional self, but RTs were the most vulnerable, given their more technical work on the floor. This was underscored when they spoke cynically about the futile attempts of the occupation to upgrade their educational requirements for credentialing and licensing. Working alone performing technical tasks did not integrate RTs into the collaborative teamwork ideal enshrined through the hospital culture.

The experience of RTs and their subdued response was also similar, at least partially, to nurses, whose work also involves technical activities prone to deskilling. Yet what positioned nurses slightly differently when it came to teamwork was their central role as coordinators of care.[8] This, in turn, countered some of the scant collaboration so prevalent among RTs, because nurses were expected to "talk" to other practitioners, to hold more extensive knowledge and skill sets in total patient care, and to be continuously visible and available at the bedside. While nurses undoubtedly experienced the contradictions between their professional aspirations, the teamwork ideal, and their work on the floor, they nonetheless exercised more leverage vis-à-vis other practitioners than did RTs, who—because of their position at the bottom of the occupational status hierarchy—may not even be considered part of the team at all.[9]

Teamwork: An Imperfect Ideal

The vignettes above provide snapshots of how the professional self fits within the organization of Hospital General, each illustrating how the hospital culture of teamwork contrasted with practitioners' conceptions of professionalism, especially regarding issues of autonomy and control. The hospital culture portrayed teamwork as a "true collaboration of equals" or as a "partnership of colleagues." But, on the floor, physicians monopolized authority, which other practitioners tried to usurp rather than resigning themselves to being marginal players following orders. Teamwork actually resembled more a collection of independent contractors than equal collaborators, especially with one member "calling the shots." Some might argue this is how it should be—that health-care teams need a leader and that it ought to be a physician.[10] It was a bitter pill to swallow, however, for most of the practitioners I spoke with.

Because the teamwork ideal supports the leading role of physicians, organizational control operates to the degree that everyone embraces it; teamwork, then, becomes ideological at the point where power relations are obscured, or at least rendered legitimate.[11] The authority vested in physician knowledge and diagnostic skills is what frequently subverts the spirit, if not the practice, of teamwork, as interoccupational conflicts left most practitioners with the short end of the stick.[12] Typically, however, I found that teamwork operated imperceptibly in patient care, other than in the exceptional cases of collaboration such as, perhaps, in the ER. Otherwise, teamwork was characterized by sequential and isolated practitioner inter-actions with each other and with patients, and it was mediated through technology such as telephones, computers, and patient charts. Such physi-cal separation enabled practitioners to enact their roles independently, thus tempering the extent to which the teamwork ideal threatened the profes-sional self. But this also had the effect of reinforcing the hierarchy, or social distance, of practitioners, whereby professional jurisdictions could remain fundamentally intact and fortified.

While physician authority remains hegemonic, the teamwork ideal may reflect some doubts about their power, given the expertise of other practitioners and the organization of health care.[13] As the vignettes show, physicians had to "hear" others' opinions, even if they objected to what they heard, in the same way they had to accept organizational directives with which they often disagreed (as I was frequently told in interviews and informal conversations). Physicians may exercise relative autonomy in the hospital, but the question is *how* relative and *how* autonomous? This con-tinuum is shaped not only by hospital management, HMOs, government programs, and peer review boards, but also by other practitioners on the team, even if these voices are heard less frequently and with less legitimacy than the teamwork ideal celebrates.

Likewise, if teamwork inadequately characterizes the underlying ten-sions in the social relations of health-care provision, it is nonetheless central to how caring is (not) organized among practitioners and within Hospital General. As I noted in the previous chapter, the teamwork ideal subsumes caring as the responsibility of "the team" and therefore actually masks its subordinate status to holding expert knowledge and curative interventions. But ideologically, the relationship of teamwork and caring operates at yet another critical level that I expand on more fully in the chapters to follow. Specifically, to be caring is to not bicker with one another, to put petty (professional) rivalries aside for the good of the patient, and *to be a team player!* In this context, teamwork serves as a symbolic glue that bonds the occupational hierarchy of professionalism I have just considered with the subordinate role of caring in Hospital General to which I now turn.

Chapter 3

The Dilemma of Caring

I'm not here to hold their hand; their mom can do that.
—ONCOLOGIST

O N A rainy autumn morning, I arrived at the hospital for a twelve-hour shift on an adult medical-surgical floor specializing in transplant patients. Located in an older wing, this unit was organized circularly with patient rooms surrounding an administrative center. I was scheduled to follow Ben, one of the day shift nurses, whom I had previously met. Ben had three patients, and even though having three patients is considered a "good assignment" among most nurses, he was very busy, because transplant patients are unstable, require close monitoring, and have a complex daily routine of medications.

One of Ben's patients was Mary, a fragile, elderly lady who was to be discharged late in the day. Every time Ben entered Mary's room, his voice softened and his hands delicately touched her arms. His body supported her when she needed to get out of bed. He smiled while talking to her, their eyes meeting as he engaged her in light conversation. Time stopped when we were with Mary: Ben never rushed his nursing routines, and his beeping pager seemed to recede quietly into the background.

When it was time for Mary's discharge, her husband arrived for her. He too was old and impaired, and he struggled to help her dress. Ben took the time to help her, respecting her privacy as he packed her belongings and made sure they were ready to leave. Later that day, Ben told me how Mary reminded him of his grandmother and how important it was to care for her as best he could. Not just physically, "not just doing the medical stuff," he said, "but caring for her at another level . . . maybe emotionally."

As I left the hospital that evening, I decided to use the main lobby rather than one of the back doors leading to the parking lot. With its shiny floors and fake plants, the lobby seemed unusually busy for the time of day. As I approached the double doors of the main entrance, trying to dodge incoming traffic, a path gradually opened around me. Slowing down, I realized that what had caused people to move aside was a patient and a nurse walking very slowly, as if in slow motion. The patient was a fragile, elderly man, wearing the staple washed-out light green gown, hunching over a walker to take one halting step at a time. He was hooked to an IV, his legs bruised, his hair thinning and white, his pale and wrinkled face looking down at the floor. I was so close to him I could see his exertions; his breathing was seriously belabored. By his side, a tall, middle-aged nurse in scrubs was pushing his IV pole and watching him. When she bent down to ask "Are you doing okay?" the man almost imperceptibly nodded his head. Noting the nurse's confident walk and calm expression, I wondered what she was thinking as they negotiated the world of fast-walking people.

In that moment, it seemed as if the buzz around me had stopped, and I found myself slowing down my own steps as they passed by me on their way out. I watched her carefully hold his right arm as the automatic doors opened and as they inched toward a bench. She moved the IV pole around him as he delicately settled onto the bench. After releasing the IV pole, she sat down, about half a foot away. They sat quietly together, as if there was no need to say or do anything other than to breathe the fresh air and gaze out into the distance. As I rejoined the world of the fast-walking people passing them by, they both smiled at me, and I thought back to Mary and how Ben had cared for her and her husband. Yet what most interested me was what it meant for Ben, and others, to practice caring this way.

When I asked practitioners about caring, they uniformly emphasized its importance in helping the sick and the vulnerable. Yet, compared to how the practitioners had discussed professionalism, I noticed a reticence and brevity as they spoke about caring, even after much probing. Over time, it seemed as if caring was indeed an ideal that, much like Ben's pager, seemed to be receding into the background of Hospital General. The discourse of caring common to practitioners involved two main dimensions that were significantly disparate for different groups: emotive and moral. The scholarship on caring has basically focused on what I am calling "emotive" caring in contrast to the dominant cure orientation in the field of medicine.[1]

Like icing put on a cake to make it look nice, emotive caring was a desirable addition to the biomedical diagnosis and curative interventions that dominated the professional ethos of all practitioners, and yet, by their own admission, it always held a lower (if not the lowest) priority in their work. But the "cure" versus "care" dichotomy shared by the practitioners I spoke with *artificially separated two interconnected spheres* of their work, which reproduced the occupational status hierarchy of Hospital General. And while physicians, nurses, and respiratory therapists alluded to this separation, they struggled to reconcile the spheres in ways that might resolve the imbalance between professionalism and caring. In contrast, OPS therapists and social workers most frequently integrated emotive caring with curing, seeing it as critical to patient recovery and well-being. Nonetheless, this proved to be the most challenging aspect of their jobs and their negotiations within the occupational status hierarchy.

Though this cure-care dichotomy was quite salient among the practitioners, they also engaged in a moral discourse that framed the dilemma of caring in a new light for me. At a basic level, an irony characterizes how the practitioners discussed caring: how can emotive caring rank so low in status and priority when all the practitioners considered it a moral aspect of health-care work? The answer lies in whether caring is framed *as an individual virtue or one that is organizationally supported.* While the former is routinely noted, the latter is notably not routine. The failure to recognize this renders caring an almost "superhuman" feat that confounds practitioners while absolving Hospital General of organizationally supporting emotive (health) care.

The Emotive Dimension

When practitioners (men and women alike) discussed caring, it was frequently as a personality trait more common to women than men. They used terms such as "emotional," "nurturing," "empathetic," "compassionate," "supportive," and even "spiritual." These characterizations are not surprising, given the concept's gendered connotations, and they resonate squarely with feminist scholarship on caring.[2] Practitioners across groups also recognized that caring could be "taught and learned," albeit with difficulty, in which case it was viewed not as genuine and sincere but rather as a deliberate act for the benefit of patients. Even respiratory therapists, the most technically oriented of the groups, emphasized the importance of an authentic personal connection when they described the emotive dimension of caring. As Dylan explained, patients will see through artificial caring and think, "Oh, he doesn't care." Dylan stressed that a caring practitioner is someone who "sees the patient with compassion and empathy." Jennie, an OPS therapist, spoke of having a "special connection" with patients, while Mike, a nurse, emphasized being someone "who patients feel they can relate to and don't feel like they're being dismissed." Dr. North, like many of his colleagues, recognized the importance of emotive caring in helping patients "not only in a medical sense but in a more psychological, emotional sense . . . to help you cope with what you are going through. But that means then that they have to be open to listen to what you have to say—someone who truly listens to the patient. . . . We would be making lots of progress medically if we did that." Sally, like her colleagues in social work, used a similar language to describe emotive caring: "It is the 'GEW' [*pronounced 'goo'*]: genuineness, empathy, warmth. . . . We should be able to be genuine in our feelings with patients. We should be empathetic with them, and we should be warm and affectionate to them. . . . This should happen in every interaction and with every person, without exception. . . . It's really about being with a patient at a different level emotionally where you understand each other that way."

After speaking with practitioners about caring, however, it quickly became evident that, with the exception of social workers and OPS therapists, they generally did not prioritize this emotive dimension as much as biomedical interventions and health outcomes. That is, the practitioners commonly referred to emotive caring but generally placed less significance on it, much as feminists have argued that behaviors or traits associated with femininity rather than masculinity are devalued and held in lower regard. As an adult oncologist dryly said, "I'm not here to hold their hand; their mom can do that. . . . Also, we're not a mental hospital or a counseling service. . . . Diagnosis and treatment—that's what we [physicians] do, and that is how we should spend our time and efforts."

This stark declaration, however, did not represent the ambivalence felt by many physicians, nurses, and RTs, and it is here that the gender framework breaks down, or is at least modified by circumstance. For example, Dr. Thompson asserted that caring is "not something we mostly are interested in or can pursue," but also explained that "I don't think it is that doctors are not caring people, I think it is that they are pushed to the point where there are so many things that they need [to do], so they put that [caring] as being low priority. . . . It's just hard with the heavy workloads we have and the fact that we are here to cure disease and illness." Indeed, while they were in the minority, several physicians mentioned the emotive side of caring despite their remoteness from the bedside and their relative insulation from prolonged patient contact in the hospital.[3] One doctor said, "If you are caring, then you really put [in] all your best effort. . . . If you really care, then you communicate with your patient and you say, 'This is what I'm going to do and let's see what happens and then you know I'm still here for you.' Especially some types of patients, like chronically ill children . . . you get better results in terms of their health outcomes."

This is not surprising, given growing concerns about the ethics of medical science; the stereotype of physicians as emotionally detached, disengaged, or uncompassionate; and a developing body of health literature valuing the emotional connection in the patient-practitioner relationship for more effective treatment and health outcomes.[4] As trends in medical schools to teach bedside manners and the basics of patient-physician interactions attest, physicians are increasingly facing institutional pressure to practice emotive caring with their patients, even at Hospital General.[5] Still, for many, this really "gets in the way of being a competent doctor" and "is not part of what physicians are supposed to do, because others are there to do it." Other practitioners were similarly conflicted about emotive caring. As Don, a veteran respiratory therapist, reflected:

> It's not easy being sick, not easy being in an ICU bed or any bed in the hospital, not knowing what the outcome might be. . . . Sometimes I think they [patients] just need to know that somebody in the hospital can be friendly—someone who is there to talk, and [to] be there for them instead of just bringing them water and then leaving. . . . But I just don't have time to do that kind of stuff! Even if I wanted [to]! The bottom line is that I'm not here to do that [caring], but I'm here to give medical treatments and improve their [patients'] physical condition.

Frequently, practitioners were called to see a patient only to discover them needing consoling rather than any specific treatment. Adam and I were chatting one day on the orthopedics floor when a nurse interrupted us, saying that one of her patients "wanted respiratory therapy," to which his doctors had agreed.

"So," Adam asked, "what's the deal with this guy?"

"I don't really know why he wants an RT," the nurse replied, "but the docs are still here so you can talk to them." Apparently, the patient had been working with a saw when his sleeve got caught and the machine "chewed up" his fingers and hand. After a long surgery to save as much of the hand as possible and to perform some reconstruction, the patient was sent to the floor for recovery.

After reading the patient's chart, Adam abruptly closed it and looked at me in disbelief. "I really don't know what we're doing here," he sighed, shaking his head. "I better talk to the docs before they leave the floor because otherwise you can't ever find them."

Spotting two physicians at a nurse's station, Adam leaned on its counter and said, "I was wondering what exactly is the problem with Mr. Knopff, 'cause I just looked at his chart and couldn't find any respiratory issues."

"Well, he said he needed it, so we put the request in," one physician replied. "Have you seen him already?"

"No," said Adam, "I just wanted to talk to you guys before I went in to make sure I know what's going on." The conversation continued for a few more minutes when it became clear that the physicians wanted Adam to go and see the patient.

After finding the room, Adam knocked on the open door and entered without waiting for a response. The nurse we had previously spoken with was talking with Mr. Knopff as we approached the bed. Adam introduced himself (and me) and then asked the nurse if the patient was on oxygen or "anything like that," to which the nurse said no. Adam asked Mr. Knopff questions about his breathing and whether he had had any respiratory illnesses in the past, and then he listened to his lungs.

"Well, Mr. Knopff," Adam said, "I am not sure you need me. I don't see you having any trouble breathing, you are talking with no difficulties, and you don't need oxygen, so I don't think I'm your guy."

Clearly upset, Mr. Knopff responded that he thought he needed respiratory therapy and he curtly told Adam that "after all I've been through, I shouldn't have to explain why I need this. It's your job, isn't it?"

Adam calmly but firmly explained that his assessment did not justify respiratory therapy but that he would talk to the doctors again. The patient mumbled an angry "OK" as we walked out.

Adam flagged the physicians, who were just about to leave the unit, and Adam informed them that he had visited Mr. Knopff and did not see any need for respiratory therapy at the moment. He asked if they knew whether he had "a history of asthma or any need at all," to which the physicians simply answered, "No, he doesn't."

After a few more minutes of discussion, Adam said decisively that there was no need for respiratory therapy and that he would formally document it. "I've told him this," Adam noted, "but you need to tell him."

The physicians nodded as they left, but Adam wanted to make sure that "everyone was on the same page," so he briefly talked to Mr. Knopff's nurse, "just in case." She repeatedly told Adam that she "got it" and that she did not understand why the physicians had requested the order in the first place. "Don't worry," she continued, "this guy [the patient] wants the attention, and he's needy. He keeps calling me and asking for this and that. He wants people to come and see him." Lowering her voice and looking around to make sure no one else was listening, she confided that "he just wants everybody to be on top of him as if he's the only one around, so I think he's definitely having some emotional issues—anxiety, stuff like that." Adam agreed and told her he had documented everything.

As we walked to another patient's room, Adam emphatically told me that "unfortunately I'm not there in the first place to be someone's psychologist or to hold their hand." What mattered most was that "whatever was physically broken gets fixed," and that was the "first priority." Later that day, while taking a short coffee break, we continued discussing this, and he again stated that his role was to give people respiratory therapy. Putting an end to the issue, he said, "If, in addition, I can help them feel like they're cared for, great, but otherwise this is not my problem or my role."

Nurses similarly found emotive caring a troubling balancing act that frequently left them with unsatisfying choices. As Kelley explained, caring required them to do *extra* work:

> Being a caring nurse means to go above and beyond your routine tasks. . . . Doing the little things that patients remember and the things that will make them feel better, like bringing them iced water

or a warm, wet washcloth even if they didn't ask, or a cup of tea when they don't expect it . . . *all those extras things that are not part of care* but help them feel and do better overall—I mean, physically better. (Emphasis added.)

Another nurse defined a caring practitioner as

somebody who really *goes out of their way* to do things for the patient, to make things personal for the patient, *beyond what you are really supposed to do.* . . . You would see somebody who makes sure that the patient's needs are met before they leave the room—*all the little extra things.* For example, if you turn off the TV when you go in to interview or work with a patient, you make sure that the TV is on before you leave the room. Or you make sure to ask if the patient needs anything before you leave the room. Even something simple like making sure they can reach their box of tissues if they have trouble moving. (Emphasis added.)

That nurses should feel that such acts are "not part of caring" but still *help* (patients) *feel better*—that they should view "all the little extra things" that meet patient needs as "beyond what you are really supposed to do"— highlights their ambivalence surrounding emotive caring and its secondary status to what they consider their primary concerns.

On another day in the medical-surgical unit, I was assigned to follow Lizzy. With five patients under her wing, she initially showed little interest in having me around. It was a nightmare shadowing her as she visited rooms distant from each other, responded to patient calls on her beeper, made phone calls to doctors and physical therapists, prepared medications, emptied bedpans, and sprinkled salt on patients' food. Focusing all of my energy, mental and physical, on attempting to keep pace with her left me exhausted within the first few hours of the shift—and Lizzy got busier as the day progressed. Having fallen behind in her charting, she barely took a break for lunch.

I noticed she was growing anxious and concerned about not having time for everything she needed to do. Before entering one of her patient's rooms, she whispered to me, "I don't have time to deal with this needy patient today; she wants so much attention and hand-holding." She continued, "They all seem really needy today." Lizzy just could "not think of doing anything else beyond the basic stuff. . . . Some days it's just a drag and today is one of those." She sighed, shaking her head, "I just don't have the time or the mental energy to hold their hand."[6]

It was clear that Lizzy had no time to chat, sit at the bedside, or console the teenager with a painful broken leg (though she administered pain medication as often as he needed it). Neither could she listen to the forty-year-old patient's wife who was in tears about her husband's surgery, nor did she have a minute to spare for Mrs. Hulloway, whose depression and anxiety were getting worse. Lizzy was overwhelmed and she could not be the "caring nurse" everyone wanted her to be. "On days like these," she lamented, "I have to prioritize and make sure they are OK physically, 'cause that is the most important thing."

For Lizzy, as for most of the nurses I observed on the floor, time was of the essence in practicing emotive caring. Because they were the first responders, they frequently faced immediate issues or dealt with emerging situations. Even for the most savvy and experienced of nurses, workload and staffing issues strained their ability to meaningfully connect with patients and their families. Nina, another nurse, indicated that emotive caring is frequently passed on to others. She recalled the case of a young patient:

> It took a lot of pain medicine just to keep him comfortable. . . . [I wondered,] "What is going on with this kid in that he needs all of these medicines?" . . . It was all anxiety driven. . . . Here these people [the physicians] had been treating his pain [physically], when it was all an emotional need. What he needed was somebody to talk to. . . . I really couldn't spend the time talking to him, but at least I was able to get a social worker in to see him. . . . At least I was able to do that!

While Nina fortunately found a social worker (i.e., a member of the group most likely—and expected—to care emotively) for this patient, nurses commonly found nobody when they looked for help in similar situations. Because nurses felt overwhelmed by immediate bedside needs, emotive caring remained up for grabs; caring was simultaneously everyone's and nobody's territory (with the exception of the understaffed and overextended social workers). Yet this hardly reflects how torn nurses were about having to choose between caring and curing. Nor did it reflect, as Sioban Nelson and Suzanne Gordon amply document in *The Complexities of Care*, how much nurses still believe in the ideal of emotive caring as part of their occupational mandate. Nor did this impugn their desire or their efforts to perform emotive caring. But if emotive caring was the "icing on the cake," nurses found it hard to spread around.

Finally, as Lizzy's shift illustrates, a key factor shaping nurses' ability to perform caring was their ultimate focus on and responsibility for providing physical treatment. Here, my observations concur with Nelson and Gordon's: while nurses at Hospital General embraced a *discourse* of emotive caring, their *actions* systematically contradicted their words. Physical intervention was a priority for nurses, and it was obvious that emotive caring was of secondary concern.[7] A post-anesthesia nurse whom I observed extensively explained why the body came first:

> I will tell you right here, right now, I want that nurse that doesn't have the great bedside manners [i.e., seems uncaring] over the one that has the great bedside. It's like when you go to your doctor—I don't care how great his bedside manner is! I want a doctor who is on the ball and knows what he is going to be doing for me. . . . If you see somebody who doesn't have that [i.e., a caring manner], I don't think that's for me to step up to them and say, "Nurse Nancy, you need to be a little more compassionate with this patient." But if they are not performing the task that they need to be doing, then I definitely do not have a problem standing up and saying, "You know what? You need to be treating their heart rate, and you need to be treating the blood pressure, you need to be treating their pain." The caring stuff comes later, and if you can do it, fine, but otherwise it is not a priority.

As the "it's not for me to step up and say" mindset illustrates, emotive caring remained a private, personal matter that defied any standardized, rule-bound procedures; that is, something that was deployed based on individual discretion. This again may not be surprising, given how caring was defined at the larger organizational level and in the workshops practitioners were encouraged to attend (see Chapter 4). Interestingly, I never witnessed conflicts over someone appearing "non-caring" at the bedside. Most of the nurses I met cautiously avoided calling someone out on this issue, although they were likely to speak up when they thought others were incorrectly intervening physically or biomedically. Here, the teamwork ideal could not operate any better in obscuring the collective responsibility of caring without holding any one practitioner responsible for (not) performing it. In this way, the caring ideal is reinforced insofar as judgments of it not being performed are rarely if ever offered. Likewise, as we will see, when practitioners refrained from criticizing colleagues, they were also absolving themselves of not living up to the moral discourse of caring they all upheld.

I found emotive caring more common among OPS therapists and social workers, compared with nurses, respiratory therapists, and physicians. This interoccupational difference was best conveyed by Wendy, a social worker:

> I see social workers as tying everything together, looking at the person as a whole and truly caring for patients . . . but they [physicians, nurses, RTs] really are centering on the physical health of that person, and once that physical health is taken care of, it's somebody else's issue to work with the emotional, psychological, or . . . the spiritual, so this isn't their problem. I think sometimes they think we're just a nuisance to have around. . . . We do "that caring stuff" and they don't really think much of it.

Social workers and OPS therapists regularly performed emotive caring in their therapeutic encounters with patients and families. The social workers I spoke with did not deny the importance of the physical treatment patients needed, but they also held that emotive caring was equally significant for patients' health recovery. OPS therapists similarly insisted that successful physical treatment required actively integrating caring in their therapeutic work.

During my research, I repeatedly observed social workers and OPS therapists—unlike physicians, nurses, and RTs—trying to help patients deal with the emotional repercussions of their physical conditions; that is, showing patients how their emotional and psychological experiences affected their recovery, and how effective therapy relied on trust and a strong relationship between practitioner and patient/family. One social worker explained that a caring social worker is "in a supportive role, in which their job is to "keep the communication going" and "to do as much as you can to help people with what they need. You know, they [patients and their families] might need something to calm them down if they're grieving—sometimes [it] is as simple as a cup of water or something like that. . . .

Sometimes it's even finding them money to buy a bus ticket or getting a meal voucher for a family member."

Although I frequently saw social workers and OPS therapists coping with time constraints and heavy workloads, I learned that these two groups did not separate emotive caring from their daily work. I first met Ellen, a physical therapist, in her department, shortly after she had received her shift assignment. First on her list was continuing therapy with a patient who had recently had a double hip replacement. Ellen knocked gently on the door; hearing a hesitant "Yes?," we entered to find a teary-eyed middle-aged woman on the bed. The blinds were still closed and her breakfast tray lay untouched on her side table.

After Ellen greeted Ms. Sealy and introduced me, the patient offered a shy smile and a restrained "good morning." Approaching the bed, Ellen asked Ms. Sealy how she was feeling, to which Ms. Sealy responded with sobs: the previous night had been terrible, she did not want to do physical therapy because she feared the pain, and she was afraid of never walking again.

After Ms. Sealy had calmed down, Ellen pulled up a chair to sit next to the bed. Ellen looked at Ms. Sealy in the eyes and softly placed her hand on the patient's forearm. "I know how you must feel. It's not easy to be in the hospital all by yourself and having had this surgery," Ellen said consolingly. "But, you know what? I am here to help you and I'm going to explain everything to you, step by step, and you can ask me or tell me anything you need to tell me, OK?" Ms. Sealy seemed to perk up, and Ellen continued by saying how important physical therapy was for Ms. Sealy to be able to walk again. She also told the patient how much she "believed in having a positive attitude and in positive thinking," and how through the years she "had seen many patients recover from this surgery with no problems. I am confident," Ellen said in an upbeat tone, "that you will leave this hospital walking."

After approximately fifteen minutes of talking with Ms. Sealy, Ellen cheerfully asked her if she was "now ready to try to get out of bed." Ms. Sealy hesitated for a brief moment, but reluctantly nodded yes. "Wonderful! That's the right attitude, Ms. Sealy," Ellen said. She moved the chair away from the bed and grabbed a folded walker that had been resting against a wall.

"Now, Ms. Sealy, I want you to pay attention to everything I say, and I want you to rely on me for support, OK?" Ellen opened the walker and set it a foot away from the bedside.

Ms. Sealy seemed scared again, but she extended her arms and put her hands on Ellen's shoulders. With some effort, Ellen supported her successfully, and in a few minutes Ms. Sealy was on her feet and holding onto the walker. Ellen moved close to her side and put an arm around her waist. "Look at that, Ms. Sealy! You did it! Are you doing OK?" she asked enthusiastically. Ms. Sealy nodded. With Ellen cheering each "little step forward," Ms. Sealy proudly took a few tiny baby steps.

As Ms. Sealy took a break, Ellen's pager rang, and she quickly glanced at it.

"You have to go now?" Ms. Sealy asked.

"No, not yet," Ellen reassured her. "I have more time to spend with you. Don't worry about it."

After more therapy, Ellen helped Ms. Sealy walk back to the bed and get back into it. As I glanced at the clock on the wall, I realized we had been with Ms. Sealy for an hour, even though it seemed as if much less time had passed. Ellen arranged Ms. Sealy's pillows, put the covers over her legs, and asked if she wanted some water. "Yes, please," Ms. Sealy breathed. Ellen poured the water, put a straw in the plastic cup, and handed it to her.

As Ms. Sealy took little sips, Ellen praised her, saying how "great" she had done and how "everything would be fine." Ms. Sealy smiled confidently this time and tenderly grasped Ellen's hand while saying "thank you." "You're very welcome," Ellen said, reassuringly patting Ms. Sealy's hand. "Now it's time for us to go, but I want you to know that I will be coming back this afternoon again to help you walk a little more, OK?"

"Fine," Ms. Sealy sighed. "Will you be coming back tomorrow, too?"

"Yes, I'll be coming every day until you are ready and healthy to go home," Ellen said, smiling, "so you'll be seeing a lot of me."

By the time we said goodbye and walked out of the room, we had spent a significant amount of focused personal time with Ms. Sealy, an experience that contrasted sharply with my many observations of nurses, physicians, and respiratory therapists. Ellen jotted some notes on her chart, spoke with the nurse for a few minutes, and we then left the floor to go work with another patient.

Ellen's interaction with Ms. Sealy shows that because time is formally structured into the labor process of OPS therapists (and arguably that of social workers, apart from providing basic welfare assistance), they can more easily perform emotive caring work *as part of* their therapeutic interventions. This factor allowed OPS therapists and social workers to listen, "get to know," counsel, and provide emotional support more routinely than physicians, nurses, and respiratory therapists, practitioners who typically treated several patients simultaneously or sequentially without having a scheduled amount of time with them. Social workers and OPS therapists were structurally positioned to nurture the type of relationship that the caring literature argues is dismissed and devalued in health care and that proponents of the "new professionalism" argue is necessary to change the nature of the practitioner-patient dynamic (and also arguably the practitioner-practitioner relationship as well).[8] Though practitioners explained that being caring required a degree of emotional involvement, without which their daily work was meaningless, they tended to internalize this dimension rather than view it as a critical (and lacking) *organizational* feature of providing health care. Consequently, they personally bore the moral weight of (not) caring.

The Moral Dimension

For practitioners across groups, the moral discourse of caring was significant because it potentially united caring with the professional self I discussed earlier; it could cast emotive caring within the context of one's professional "calling" to serve others or the public good.

Likewise, this discourse allowed practitioners to show *to themselves* as well as others their quality as individuals; it was an expression of their virtuous character. In describing themselves as caring practitioners, they typically referred to being respectful, nonjudgmental, and humane, being good people with good intentions and honorable intrinsic qualities, and always being advocates for those they served. In the words of Thomas, a physical therapist, "If you don't care about people—if you don't care about how they feel, what they think, what they're dealing with—you're in the wrong job! You better go work on computers all day! Or something where you don't have to work with people! I'd tell people that! We're caring people—good people helping others; we are all in this because we want to do things for others who need us."

Jane, a speech therapist with many years of experience, agreed with him: "It's important for us to remember that what we're doing is important and why we're doing it. I think if you do this work and you don't care about your patients or others, then you might as well just go work in a factory!

It's about remembering that we are all good people here, working hard. . . . We're in this job because we're good-hearted people." Trent, a respiratory therapist, emphatically told me, "It is exactly why we are here! I mean, I chose this field because I do care! I like to help people." He added that caring was "the absolute—the most important—reason to be here," and that it was about "doing for others without expecting anything back" and "being a good person," reiterating that "this is who we are and this is what we do!"

Among social workers, this view of caring as a moral virtue was also typical. One practitioner said:

> Sometimes I hear from friends and relatives, "How could you work over there [in a hospital]? You work with all these drug addicts and you work with all those sick people." Everybody is a human being and I honestly believe that it's not my place to judge. I just want them [patients] to understand that we truly care about people, that we have a good heart, and that we are doing this not for ourselves but for others who need us. . . . It is not just a paycheck. We are caring people who want to do good and that takes a very special type [of individual].

Susan, another social worker, reflected that "a caring social worker is really a protector. . . . Being caring means having the good morals and the good character to advocate for the weak and do the best on their behalf."

Dr. Schuster put it this way: "We are a caring profession. Caring is beyond knowledge and skills. . . . Caring is about us being our best to help them [patients]. . . . It's really about having this strong commitment to helping others regardless of the inconveniences that [it] may personally cause us sometimes or regardless of the price you have to pay for helping others! It's about the kind of person you are."

Sharing a similar view of caring as a matter of individual virtue, another nurse discussed it in these words:

> The only thing you have with a person is the humanity of it and the honesty of it. . . . As caregivers, we want people [patients] to know that we're doing this for you [patients] because we mean well and because we went into this job to do for others and help people. . . . Taking care of patients is hard and you have to be a good person and have that motivation in your heart to guide you along. . . . I treat

people as I want to be treated: "Do unto others as you'd have them do unto you."

But most importantly, in my opinion, this moral discourse of caring emphasized deep and powerful transformations of the self in which "extraordinary" people do "extraordinary" work. The points made by Cathy, a nurse, are representative of this view:

> There are so many easier ways to make a good living! The intimacy that is required for a nurse to provide care for a patient is physical [and] emotional intimacy. You would not put yourself at that kind of risk or be that vulnerable to other people if you didn't care! Again, at some point people may experience fatigue from that, and it is important for all of us to buoy each other up and support one another through those really dry times when you feel like you don't care—when you feel you can't care even one more time, or *give yourself away one more time*. (Emphasis hers.)

Though undoubtedly admirable, emotive caring can exact a significant personal toll, and here Cathy spoke for practitioners who felt unable to give themselves away "one more time." The moral dimension of caring affirmed one's professional self, but it also ultimately threatened to *sacrifice it* to the degree that caring was internalized (i.e., understood as a personal virtue that only individuals could act on). In this sense, being a caring professional was truly a heroic act and those who were known as such shone brighter than all the rest. Indeed, listening to practitioners speak about caring, I was struck by how frequently they framed it in almost spiritual terms, especially among nurses, for whom the symbolic framework of caring harkens back to a Nightingale mythology of near-sacred proportions.

If one views caring as a heroic act, one can begin to make sense of the irony I noted at the beginning of this chapter: how can emotive caring rank so low in status and priority when all practitioners consider it a moral aspect of health-care work and of their professional selves? By definition, heroic acts are "above and beyond" what most of us are capable of in the daily routines of our lives, including in our jobs. But that does not preclude us from holding heroic ideals, for this is what the moral dimension of caring represents: an ideal that dignifies the professional self even if, by their own accounts, practitioners seldom live up to it. Equally important is the degree to which practitioners view caring as an individual virtue, for only individuals can perform heroic acts. Institutions and organizations are not heroic—people are—and if caring "is not my job" or "not what I'm here to do," it nonetheless lingers in the nether symbolic regions of practitioners' professional selves as a nagging reminder that something is missing from the provision of health care, and that something is not quite right at Hospital General.

Interestingly, OPS therapists and social workers, for whom emotive caring is more fully integrated into their work routines, are not the anomaly they might appear to be. For OPS therapists, caring is central to achieving successful recuperation, but they still emphasize physiological diagnosis and intervention. And though they enjoy a more structurally favorable situation to integrate emotive caring in treating patients, they still face working conditions (see Chapter 5) that frequently meant "not doing everything you are supposed to do in the way you're supposed to." But here, too, emotive caring constitutes a personal challenge, not organizational neglect.

Likewise, social workers overwhelmingly emphasize emotive caring, and their discourse of the morality of caring has deep roots in the birth of social work at the turn of the twentieth century. Most early social workers worked in urban slums or as "charity" workers commissioned by state agencies to look after the poor and disenfranchised as government joined private philanthropy and religious institutions in providing public welfare.[9] But the social justice orientation of advocacy and protectionism is not as ascendant today as the clinical wing in social work, and even if social workers uphold this ideological strand of their occupational heritage, theirs is still a marginal voice that is unlikely to redefine heroic caring in Hospital General.

Finally, this pervasive focus on the morality of caring as an individual virtue runs the risk of neglecting practitioner-practitioner as well as practitioner-patient relations—something that scholarship on caring and the "new professionalism" frames as requiring deep social and institutional transformations to arrive at more just work arrangements, more egalitarian relationships with patients, and a more equitable society in general.[10] If caring is viewed as an individual virtue, it does not transcend social hierarchies; instead, it reinforces the elite status of professionals by narrowing the parameters of what constitutes valued knowledge while failing to mend the artificial separation of the care-cure dichotomy I noted earlier. Rather than being central to the professional self and organizationally supported, caring remains concealed within a discourse of teamwork that disregards the occupational status hierarchy.

This ideology of caring reaffirms a normative order in which practitioners must always be "good," even under the most difficult circumstances. They must constantly ignore or avoid any negative feelings and desires they may have vis-à-vis other practitioners and patients alike, for clearly such attitudes contradict the image of a health-care team devoted to the best patient care. This is why the caring workshops I describe in the following chapter are so ideological—they promote just this obfuscation of the status hierarchy. The penalties for violating such moral expectations are high, ranging from a personal sense of not belonging to guilt in not seeing beyond "mundane" workplace issues, informal sanctioning by those in higher ranks, coworkers' disapproval, and even the potentially loss of one's job. And this is also why sanctions against noncaring practitioners are never made public, as it would risk tearing away the ideological veil of caring. As ideology, caring sanctifies practitioners' experiences and professional relations, and it may very well be the fragile bond that holds the entire edifice together. Yet this fragility underscores the dilemma faced by practitioners in the organization of health care, and it alerted me to another discourse of caring—one that was not fully articulated by practitioners but was still pervasive in Hospital General. I now turn to considering how caring also constitutes a form of resistance to the dehumanizing aspects of institutional life.

Chapter 4

Caring Reconsidered

Caring for others helps you get through the day.
—REGISTERED NURSE

ARAH, a petite woman and a senior nurse, had impressed me with her multitasking skills and her energy as she moved across the cardiac unit from one patient to another. Around lunchtime, a fellow nurse asked if she wanted anything, to which Sarah responded, "Yeah, get me a large lemonade; I'll give you the money when you come back."

"No problem," the other nurse said. "By the way, can you keep an eye on my guy in 32 until I get back? You don't have to worry about the others—two of them are not here and the other one just got back from a procedure and she's totally asleep."

A few minutes later, Sarah was asked to report to the nurses' station. There, Ruth told her that Mr. Hayes in 32 was calling "again." "He's been on the call light the whole morning," Ruth sighed, rolling her eyes and shaking her head.

Upon arriving at Mr. Hayes' room, we were greeted with a mouthful of discontent: "I have been calling you guys; I've been waiting for this or the other the whole morning!"

I was immediately taken aback and felt very uncomfortable, but Sarah never broke stride. "Hello, Mr. Hayes, do you remember me?" she responded calmly. "I took care of you last week, and I met your wife and daughter, too." Smiling, Sarah approached his bed and softly placed her hand on his shoulder as she glanced at his IV. She then patted his hand, and Mr. Hayes' angry frown softened.

"What can I do for you today?" she asked, in a reassuring tone. "How can I help you?"

"Well, I asked the gal who's with me today for something for my lips— you know, some Vaseline or something—because they are so chapped! You see, they are bleeding, and I asked her like two hours ago, and nothing . . ."

"Oh, no, I'm so sorry you didn't get that sooner, but I'll go and get it for you right away and we'll take care of those lips. Don't you worry, I'll be right back."

Mr. Hayes thanked Sarah with a smile. Upon returning with the Vaseline, Sarah helped him apply it.

"All better now, Mr. Hayes?" she asked, once again placing her hand on his shoulder.

"Yes, that's all I needed, you see. Thank you," he responded.

Sarah told him that he could call any time if he needed something and that she would let his current nurse know about this.

Sarah continued attending to her other patients, but we never heard back from Mr. Hayes. About half an hour later, as we sat in the break room while Sarah charted, I asked her about Mr. Hayes and his mood. "If you put in a few caring minutes with somebody," Sarah explained, "it sure makes your day easier. . . . One of my favorite things to do is [to] walk in on a belligerent patient like that and put them at ease. Showing that you care makes your day easier, because once you establish that rapport with somebody, then it's just a breeze. . . . It's a more pleasant interaction and it makes my day better! And, of course, it makes his day better, too."

Frequently, practitioners spoke of how it "had been proven" that caring (i.e., being attentive to patients, communicating with them, letting them know that one has their best interest at heart, and satisfying small requests immediately) led to happy patients and speedier recovery. In the words of an RT, "happy patients are more understanding and willing to cut you some slack." Patients experienced various problems related to time delays in care, lack of information, and feeling they were not cared for properly. These patient complaints corresponded closely with findings I reviewed in the hospital's patient satisfaction surveys, which were systematically conducted after patients were discharged.[1] In short, the common refrain on the floor was that fewer "needy" or disgruntled patients meant fewer conflicts. Being an outsider, I felt much less uncertainty and insecurity when patients were friendly with me, and I came to see how this could also be the case for nurses, RTs, OPS therapists, and social workers, who frequently used caring to ease the course of interactions between them and those they helped. As a speech therapist aptly put it:

> I think it's very important. For me, I don't think I could get very much done if you're not caring. The patients can sense that you don't really care—that you just want to get in and get out and do your thing because you're busy and have other patients and things to do. . . . But *if you can find a way of being caring that they can see or sense,* they will respond to you the way you treat them, and then you can get things accomplished more easily. (Emphasis added.)

This example of what Arlie Hochschild calls "deep acting" (a more authentic practice than "surface acting," which is the performance of artificial displays in order to keep a job) exacts an emotional toll on practitioners, as I documented in the previous chapter; this is another reason why I identify it as heroic and virtuous.[2] It is also possible, however, that caring operates at another level that supports and expands on Hochschild's analysis of emotional labor. As part of the health-care labor process (though neglected or of lower priority), caring is subject to exploitation, and arguably more so than labor that is considered more cognitively based.[3] Though all practitioners deploy cognitively based skills, some skill sets, such as those associated with caring, are less valued than others.[4]

As Daniel Chambliss argued in *Beyond Caring,* caring operates within a powerful ideological field as a point of contention in the health-care workplace, especially insofar as nurses consider it a symbolic measure of their moral superiority over physicians.[5] But I rarely observed conflict between practitioners over who did or did not perform caring, nor did nurses define their professional self exclusively in this way. Rather, the ideological character of caring is more salient at an organizational level, where it (alongside the teamwork ideology I discussed in Chapter 2) implicates the characteristically alienating and dehumanizing experience of what Erving Goffman in *Asylums* termed a "total institution."[6] Likewise, given that cure and care work are subject to exploitation in a market-based (or nationalized) system of health-care delivery, the ideology of caring may function to conceal, or at least rationalize, how practitioners experience such exploitation. The caring I observed and practitioner discourse about caring can both be viewed as *acts of resistance* to these features of health care in the United States.

Framed in this way, caring can also be understood ideologically as promoting authentic and sincere social relationships within a larger institutional terrain of struggle.

Caring as Ideology

As my fieldwork evolved, I became intrigued by how much organizational emphasis was placed on the issue of caring. I collected various printed materials, such as pamphlets and flyers, that were available throughout the hospital. This material stated how Hospital General and its practitioners were committed to a caring environment and practice. In a local television advertising campaign to promote the hospital's health-care services, a nifty slogan portrayed it as providing top-quality care for "the heart and the soul." Walking through the hallways (particularly near the main lobby, where there was heavy patient and practitioner traffic), one could find large, colorful, shiny, and eye-catching posters about "caring." The posters mostly provided information about how caring had a positive impact on patient health outcomes as well as on the working environment. In short, Hospital General devoted considerable resources to publicizing its commitment to caring, as if it were part of its competitive edge in the region.

At another level, junior physicians in training were offered "doctoring" classes to sharpen their medical skills and to learn how to treat patients in a compassionate and humane way. Likewise, senior and attending physicians were occasionally invited to workshops on how to positively interact, communicate, and empathize with patients. These workshops and conferences were held at the hospital and emphasized the importance of understanding, establishing a relationship, and "connecting" with patients. These events were not mandatory, and I learned they were poorly attended by higher-ranking physicians, while interns and residents went more frequently. "Many of us just don't show up," an attending surgeon told me on our way to the operating room. "It's like a joke! I don't need to sit there to listen to someone tell me how to be with my patient." Other occupations also had their versions of these workshops—"in-services," as they were called—which covered similar topics.[7]

Perhaps the best example I encountered of this organizational effort to promote caring was a two-day nursing staff workshop contracted by the hospital administration out to an independent consulting firm, Future Care

Incorporated (FCI).[8] Attendance was not mandatory, but I observed on the floor that nurse managers encouraged nursing staff to go, because they believed it was beneficial. The workshop ran from eight in the morning to four in the afternoon, and it was directed by a group composed of FCI's vice president, the nursing assistant director, the primary nursing manager, and a few nurses who had been trained in FCI's philosophy and techniques. Each participant was assigned to a group of eight to ten individuals who were supposed to become one's "family" for the workshop. The atmosphere was relaxed, people wore regular clothes instead of scrubs, and meditation music played softly in the background. The groups sat at large round tables where paper, coloring pencils, watercolors, brushes, and other "creative" materials had been placed. Snacks and drinks were readily available throughout the day, along with a catered breakfast and lunch. Afternoon coffee was served with expensive baked goods such as gourmet French pastries.

Some workshop activities focused on helping nurses get in touch with their "spirit," with the "soul of nursing," and with "genuine caring." The FCI vice president spoke about "the need for nurses to feed the spiritual and return to the Nightingale model that's been lost," "the need to go back to primary nursing," and, above all, "remembering that [nursing] is a call from God." Other tasks were targeted at "connecting" staff with each other at an emotional level so they might better understand what makes patients feel good. For example, one exercise required that we choose a partner at our table and give them a hand massage for five minutes. We were then asked to discuss how it felt and what it meant to us.

Another set of activities instructed participants on how to create "positive" working relations with staff and how to resolve "issues" one might have with other nurses or practitioners. The principles guiding all the group participation, videos, written material, and open discussions emphasized building a consensus around "being happy with your job." For example, one of these materials was a pocket-size "embracing my colleagues" booklet, which focused on establishing relationships of trust with other staff based on respect and without "whining, finger-pointing, and backstabbing." In keeping with such affirmations, other activities reinforced being accountable for one's actions and work performance. Likewise, participants were advised about the "power of patients" in shaping nurses' work experiences.

We were reminded to "never tell patients you will do something that then you do not do" and to "always remember that you are treating patients' families too." We were repeatedly told that "patients love their nurses," that "each nurse is a unique individual," and that "you, as a nurse, have the power to change others, one smile at a time." This was, as FCI's vice-president stated at the conclusion of the workshop, "the most important contribution of the new sciences focusing on the power of intention." The message was clear: be nice, be a good worker, serve others at all costs . . . and enjoy it.

As I left the workshop, I wondered whether the hospital had sponsored this event because caring was a "problem area" that required improvement. All of this—the posters on the walls, the hospital's television commercial, the usual conversations on the floor, and the workshops—made me question why there was so much organizational effort to promote caring. On the one hand, I had seen and heard how most practitioners struggled with or de-prioritized caring. And, if the patient satisfaction surveys showing low scores in this area were reliable in any way, it is not surprising that the hospital administration held such concerns, or that it sincerely believed in reminding practitioners to perform caring beyond their obvious mandated tasks. Still, such institutional efforts framed caring as an individual act; the onus was placed on practitioners, who were expected to practice caring with little organizational support or policies that might alleviate their already heavy working demands. Whether it expressed an inner calling or enacted a strategy for coping, caring increased practitioner workloads, since they were expected to perform it on top of everything else.

Likewise, the workshop and other organizational promotions of caring were less about reviving a calling to care than reinforcing being a "good worker," given the problems associated with occupational status differentials and labor processes in the hospital. Why would the hospital administration encourage embracing one's colleagues through a pocket-size card for the practitioners to carry around were this not a problem? Why so much emphasis on the transcendent nature of caring (i.e., "a calling from God") if profane, secular conflicts on the floor and between occupational groups were not an issue? The ideology of caring conceals these problems while providing a symbolic source of cohesion and common ground among occupational groups and the hospital administration. I am not suggesting by this that people do not sincerely care about patients. On the contrary, all the practitioners expressed strong beliefs and a predisposition to caring in diverse ways. I am questioning the necessity of this organizational effort, which requires extensive resources and is intended to motivate practitioners who *already* come to the hospital with a caring orientation. While the hospital may hope to reinforce this orientation as the reality of working in a large hospital gradually (or not) sinks in, the ideology of caring posits it as an individual virtue and responsibility rather than an obligation of larger organizational dimensions. As Ariel Ducey observed in similar "in-services" workshops in a New York City hospital, "these training programs do not address the key problems of health care work: inadequate staffing levels, expanding workloads, lack of material support, and unresponsive structures of authority. Instead, they focus on adjusting the worker to the situation."[9] Ducey later writes, "In fact, training programs arguably became the only, and therefore inevitably inadequate, response to the pressures and stresses front line workers faced."[10]

In this light, one must ask how the ideology of caring resonates in the hearts and minds of practitioners. Ideologies are frequently contested, especially when such rhetoric and symbolic appeals become transparent and reveal vested interests.[11] As I listened to practitioners talk about caring, I gradually began to hear another discourse that challenged how health care is organized at Hospital General. At times restrained and at times forceful, this more subdued yet potentially powerful discourse fundamentally held that doing care work meant confronting and resisting the alienating and dehumanizing aspects of the hospital, as well as the exploitative nature of the health-care labor process. This discourse was most common among nurses, insofar as they expressed the most ambivalence about caring, given its role in their jobs (and this was likely why they were most strongly encouraged to attend these workshops). Recall that physicians and respiratory therapists placed caring second to their primary responsibilities, with OPS therapists and social workers having it structured into their time with patients. Nurses, on the other hand, were expected to care based on occupational and historically based stereotypes, but they also struggled with time constraints, heavy workloads, and their ongoing pursuit of recognition within the health-care community (especially among their medical peers). While caring as resistance may not articulate a coherent or fully developed alternative model for health care, it nonetheless represents a critique of the health-care system. A gesture far more significant than simply

not attending a workshop, it emerges from the bedside experiences of practitioners who are acting on behalf of patient welfare toward a more humane
and just organization of health care.

Caring as Resistance

One day, in a medical-surgical unit, I followed one of the social workers,
Terri, and a nurse, Rose. One of Rose's patients suffered from an incurable
disease and had spent an extended period of time in the hospital. Rose had
cared for this woman intermittently for several months as she underwent
different treatments, hoping that they would extend her life. Every time
we entered the patient's room, it was clear that Rose and the woman had
developed a close relationship.

As the day progressed, Rose got word of her patient's latest test results,
which were dire. "I don't know what to do," she sighed. "This is so sad, and I
can't believe the doctors can't find a way of making things a little better for
her." I listened as Rose debated with herself on whether to "call the social
worker now" or "wait until after the docs have talked to her." She finally
decided to call Terri to help the woman cope with the bad news.

A while later, as we stood at the nurses' station, a group of physicians
approached Rose and said they were ready to see the patient. I decided not
to follow them, as this was clearly a private situation and there were already
too many people in the room with whom the patient had to share her grief.
Less than twenty minutes later, the physicians exited the room, speaking to
each other in hushed tones; Rose followed them out, visibly shaken, teary-
eyed, and upset. The social worker, Terri, then left the room, having told
the woman that she would return later.

In the nurses' break room, Terri sat down at one of the long tables next
to Rose. Terri put her arm around Rose and gently rubbed her back. "I
know this is hard for you," she said softly, "but we are here to care for each
other too." She continued, "I'm here not just for patients but for the staff as
well, you know."

Unexpectedly, Rose turned on her, saying she had expected Terri to talk
to the doctors before they went in. Terri looked disconcerted as Rose continued, "I can't believe you just let them tell her cold turkey like that and
then they get to walk away and we are left with the mess."

Terri momentarily removed her arm from Rose's back, but she looked

Rose in the eyes and listened intently as the agitated nurse criticized her. Then Terri placed her hand on Rose's shoulder once again, and calmly replied, "Rose, you know, we have to remember that we are all here to help—that we are all caring people. That's why we do this work. . . . I know you think I should have done something different, but right now, if we remember that, we can put our differences aside and try to do our best for this patient." Rose calmed down and nodded, even as the beeper in her pocket sounded off insistently. "Besides," Terri added, pointing to Rose's beeper, "you have other patients who need you too, and you need to take care of them, so you have to get back out there and do what you can for the others."

Rose got up, took a deep breath, and thanked Terri. They smiled at each other as we all walked out the door.

For the rest of the day, Rose attended to her patients almost as if nothing had happened. As the shift ended, and we gathered our belongings in the break room, Rose told me that it was a "good thing" that Terri had reminded her that she needed "to get back out there" and care for her other patients. "She's really caring," Rose said of Terri, "and caring for the others helps you get through the day."

"Helps you get through the day" is a refrain I heard so frequently at Hospital General. Though it was not always apparent in my interviews, practitioners used caring to cope not only with patients but also with each other and their disagreements on the floor, as this last vignette illustrates. This was just one instance among the many others I observed where a practitioner reached out to a distraught colleague in order to defuse conflicts, clarify work priorities, and give and receive encouragement throughout the day. While this affirms the ideology of care as social control ("you have to get back out there"), it also reflects practitioners resisting the frequently alienating and often dehumanizing atmosphere of Hospital General. Terri connected with Rose emotionally, even though they were only vaguely familiar with each other from working occasionally in the same unit (since social workers tended to "float" or rotate throughout the hospital). For both Terri and Rose, caring for each other as well as patients constitutes a refusal to surrender to the most disturbing aspects of a total institution.

As another nurse explained, caring can cast the status quo in doubt: "I can't tell you how many times physicians come up and they want to do something to a child and the nurse always intervenes. They think we are just "mothering" the patient, but I see it as questioning how things are done here [in the hospital]." The nurse complained that in their eagerness "to go in there and do it," physicians fail to recognize that their patients "need help with coping with what's happen[ing] to them." When, to address this, the nurses sit with patients and talk to them, the physicians "just think it's just us [nurses] doing what we do, fluffing pillows." Similarly, Rob lamented how hospital management and physicians regarded the nurses as "softies," but he insisted that "patients need more than the meds." He stated that the hospital needed to be more holistic about caring, and to provide family-centered care (such as enabling patients' families to stay with them overnight). He emphasized that its nurses had "been trying to do that for years . . . but the hospital has issues."

Caring challenged the objectification of patients, and though some may argue that a degree of this is required for effective treatment, nurses consistently held that it should not come at the expense of the humanity and dignity of patients or staff. As Claire explained: "You do the caring. . . . Number one, you look at the patient in the eye. Number two, you talk to the patient as a real person. You talk to the person as a real human being and you see that people are really interesting. . . . You ask them questions [to] find out all kinds of things about them." Another nurse shared this view, saying that the hospital and its physicians "look at the patient as a diagnosis and achievement. . . . The patient is a surgery site and that's it. . . . They [patients] want to know they are not just a number. . . . They [patients] depend on us [nurses]. They are vulnerable."

Given how disempowering and dehumanizing the hospital experience can be for patients and practitioners alike, acts of caring were often attempts to reestablish these relationships on a different ground—one where notions of justice were never far below the surface. June, a veteran of Hospital General, asserted that really caring nurses truly understand the complexity of interacting with different types of patients, and that "caring is more providing dignity and respect for that whole person—respect and dignity, because you don't get that here" in the hospital. As an example, June cited caring for a homeless man "as if he was the same as a VIP," emphasizing that at Hospital General the difference in status is pronounced. "When you do caring, you are treating all equally. They all get respected the same, [so] that the psycho patient who is calling you names, and hitting and kicking, is never degraded because of his psychosis. So I have to know how to care for all these different people." She reiterated that caring beyond the biomedical is so important in the hospital because its patients "are just a number."

Some nurses even framed caring as a way to address underlying problems such as social inequality and patient rights. In the words of one RN:

> We do the caring. . . . We have the most opportunity to bring that holistic care into the plan, 'cause everyone else [is] just dealing with the medical. But as a nurse you hear and pay attention, you sit down and have a bedside chat with the family, you ask questions with a purpose. . . . We are able to recognize needs that are ignored. . . . We deal with all of it. If the families are short on cash, [if] they have no money for food, we are the first ones to find out that there is trouble. . . . Caring is therapeutic and part of helping people who are in dire straits . . . or addressing people rights like a child's rights, or end of life rights. . . . We understand and know the how and whys of patients.

The objectification of patients as essentially biomedical entities was compounded by organizational mandates pushing the bottom line, and emotive caring offered many nurses an alternative voice that empowered them against these larger organizational forces. As another nurse explained:

> Knowing [how] to do caring, it's part of being a nurse, but you just don't do all the time or just don't do for the touchy feely stuff. . . . We [nurses] do it for a reason. . . . Mainly, you can't just be here [in the hospital] doing business. . . . Giving your meds is business. Giving them [meds] and just walking out, you can do that. But while I'm giving meds, I'm talking to the patient, to the family, so that they [patients] are not just a "thing" we do things to. . . . They [patients] are not just a business.

It is important to note that resistance through caring embodied dilemmas that put nurses between a rock and a hard place. "I think caring skills are essential for nursing," Stacey said, but she also noted that nurses sometimes feel compelled to consider "withholding the caring component." She added, however, that "this would be very difficult for the patient," so nurses end up worrying about the patient, such that the withholding might "not be as rewarding for the nurse." The dilemma of withholding caring was hard to resolve, mainly because practitioners believed in how important caring skills and caring work are for health and healing. Yet nurses in particular felt extremely conflicted about their own interests in relation to those of their patients.[12] Reflecting on this problem, Mary's comments echo those of other nurses:

> I think you can stop doing the caring stuff. . . . I have to be pretty frustrated to stop the caring. But even when I'm frustrated, you still have to care about what's being done and the progress of the patient. . . . At some basic level, you just care about that. . . . I think I'm fooling myself sometimes into not getting frustrated, because when I think about how much I have to do and what doctor I have to talk to, it can be really frustrating . . . and when that happens, nurses will usually take it out on the patient—not really wanting to, but it just happens that way. You stop the caring stuff. That's the only thing you can do sometimes. . . . At the same time, I'm here for the patient and because I want to help people, and so we [nurses] have to keep that in mind and make decisions about what to do.

Nonetheless, nurses were on guard against the more insidious ways that caring led to self-exploitation. For example, one nurse spoke of how deciding to hold back on caring is difficult but perhaps necessary, stating that "you have to know to back down." She observed that when caring nurses

> put themselves a little bit second, but not completely, then you get into this thing with too many nurses who have "Martha complexes" and that is not good for you [as a worker]. . . . You need to know when enough is enough and stop. . . . You hear them [nurses] say, "I should have gone home four hours ago, but they [patients] really need me here. . . ." I say, "Oh, please go home, they don't need you that bad. . . ." It's a slippery slope, you know.

Time was always in short supply for nurses, and if caring came up short at the day's end, it was still on their shoulders tomorrow. One practitioner spoke of having to figure out "how to focus when there is a lot of background noise in the nurse's day. I guess . . . everybody has the same amount of time in a twenty-four-hour day. How you use that time at the bedside is something that you can make some choices about . . . but it's hard."

It should be noted that, as a meaningful form of resistance at the bedside, caring does not always, or necessarily, involve pitched social conflict. As sociologists have documented for some time, resistance can take many subtle forms beyond armed rebellion or organized public protests.[13] One might also ask why caring as resistance is more common among nurses than other practitioners. Based on my analysis so far, I believe that two factors account for this. Structurally, nurses are the one group that does not enjoy what Steven Lopez terms "organized emotional care," where caring is formally integrated into their time spent with patients.[14] While physicians and respiratory therapists are not expected to provide such caring, nurses are, but without the time to deploy it, as is the case with social workers and OPS therapists. In this context, resistance emerges from a conflict between occupational aspirations and organizational expectations at the point of health-care provision. This conflict is intensified by a cultural factor, the Nightingale myth, in which emotive caring epitomizes the work of nursing. To the degree that nurses still harbor this myth (as Nelson and Gordon argue), their professional self is incomplete—stunted, so to speak—as they struggle to meet what they view as their professional calling.[15] To some extent, then, caring as resistance represents how nurses experience their work in a total institution, but it is also a defense of their professional ideals, be they mythical, idealistic, or ideological.

Despite serious obstacles, caring as resistance can nurture the building of shared interests between practitioners and with patients while cultivating alternative models of health-care delivery. But for this to occur, caring must be viewed as a collective action that is organizationally supported, not a solitary act of sincere yet physically and emotionally exhausted individuals. All practitioners face organizational pressures and constraints that threaten their professional and caring ideals alike. How do they deal with these issues on the floor? In the following chapter, I focus on what practitioners regard as the central problems of hospital work, and then explore two distinct approaches to these problems and how they ultimately fall short of unifying professionalism and caring.

Chapter 5

When the Day Is Done, It's Still Work

What we do is really hard work.
Sometimes I wonder why I'm still here.
—REGISTERED NURSE

IME, workload, staffing . . ." Jason, a respiratory therapist, exhaled in frustration as we scurried down the hall to another patient. "They have suddenly increased our workload. I know they're looking for productivity, but the more they look for productivity, the busier we are, the worse for patients. Sometimes you take shortcuts or you rush through, knowing that you are not doing the best work. . . . [At] other times, we are not charting everything that we are doing, so it is not showing up in productivity."

Jason turned around a sharp corner without even peeking at the large corner mirrors perched above it (as they were at all corridor intersections). "They say, 'Well, you are overstaffed, you don't need as many respiratory therapists.' Yet, we are going, 'How can we be overstaffed, because we are busting our asses to get everything done?' It's a never-ending cycle." Jason's beeper was sounding off as we wove frantically through oncoming staff, some glancing at their wristwatches, others with eyes focused on charts, and still others pushing or pulling large stretchers, some empty and some ferrying patients to yet another test or procedure. After a year of following various practitioners through similarly chaotic hospital traffic, I was still amazed that nobody had crashed into anyone or anything else. But then, at Hospital General, people never crashed . . . until after work.

As patients, we are seldom privy to the conditions under which practitioners toil day and night. Even those of us who have stayed in a hospital beyond a few days witness only those fragments of hospital life that come to our room or to which our illness exposes us. Yet for the health-care workers at Hospital General, there were systemic problems that, during each and every shift, tested their professional and caring ideals. These problems centered around three main issues: unfavorable working conditions, conflicts with patients and families, and, to a lesser degree, lack of adequate resources.

Practitioners' perceptions of these workplace issues are not unfounded, having been widely documented in hospitals nationwide.[1] Since the 1970s, many social scientists have argued that managed care and increasing bureaucratization of the health system have negatively impacted physician autonomy, while others hold that physicians have continued to assert control over their practice.[2] Certainly the rise of physician unions is testimony to the growing frustration felt by many in this most elite occupation.[3] And numerous studies have shown how managed care has undermined the working conditions of nurses and what Ariel Ducey calls the "allied" or "frontline" health-care workers of the sub-baccalaureate labor market.[4] When the day is done, providing care is still work even for employees in a prestigious urban hospital, be they privileged professionals or undervalued hired hands.

What follows may shed light on these debates, but my intent is to understand practitioner concerns in the wider context of the health-care division of labor. In addition to evaluating their perceptions against documented evidence (which I attempt to some degree), practitioners routinely spoke of these problems in the hospital, and as sociologist W. I. Thomas famously asserted, "If men define situations as real, they are real in their consequences."[5] How practitioners defined reality, then, served as an organizational canvas against which the professional self might be inscribed, and as a symbolic backdrop to the fate of caring in Hospital General. My discussion here bridges the previous chapters with those that follow in terms of how to understand and resolve the tensions between professionalism and caring in the context of this work atmosphere. Importantly, not all groups were equally disgruntled, because some could better avoid or fend off these issues, given the nature of their jobs and their positions in the hospital. Nor would it be accurate to say that these health-care workers did not enjoy their jobs; surely one can like a job and still bemoan its nightmares. While the accounts that follow may not resemble the tales so vividly depicted in ethnographies of working-class factory life, perhaps the modern hospital does constitute a factory of sorts for these health-care practitioners.[6]

Working Conditions

Hospital General is one of the best in the region, taking pride in high-quality and state-of-the-art patient care. Yet, after talking with practitioners, one might be startled by their discontent with the day-to-day working conditions, which included inadequate staffing, heavy workloads, and lack of time. While all the groups viewed these as chronic problems, not all expressed the same degree of concern or dissatisfaction with them. Among the practitioners I interviewed, just over half of the physicians saw working conditions as a problem, followed by a majority of the OPS therapists and nurses. In contrast, practically all the social workers and respiratory therapists I spoke with lamented their working conditions.

It Could Be Worse . . .

Running his hand through his graying yet full head of hair, Dr. Blumstein deplored the stress of understaffing. "I feel overextended, so I'm not thrilled about that," he sighed. "There is such a push to have a high census and high patient loads, and yet they [administrators] don't take into account what happens. Let's say we add three patients to our unit. Well, they add a nurse, but we don't have the attending physician staff to be able to add more attendants to the service. . . . So, we feel extended."

The administration's push to admit more patients was not the only reason physicians felt pressured. The legal requirements limiting the hours of residents were a factor. Noting the heavy workloads and long hours that impaired their ability to provide high-quality care, Dr. Whyte also alluded to the toll on physicians in general: "The busier the hospital is, the harder it is for us to provide everybody with the care that they deserve. The workload is a constant issue. . . . That's part of the reason there has been pressure on getting our [residents'] work hours down to a more reasonable level. But I do think that is part of what goes along with our fatigue and people getting burned out."

A vicious cycle had become institutionalized, where hospital demands to increase patient admissions (a key source of profit) exacerbated inadequate staffing due to occupational shortages, poor retention, and turn-over—conditions further complicated by external legal regulations (e.g., residents' work hour regulations and medical malpractice concerns). Physicians routinely spoke of how burnout and stress undermined the quality of their work and taxed their sense of professional calling.[7] As one surgeon lamented, "Try being on call and having to come in at the drop of a hat at three in the morning!" Yet, for most, it seemed this was just part of the job—perhaps a Faustian bargain for elite status on the health-care team. As one descends the occupational hierarchy, however, this bargain recedes amid increasing concerns over working conditions.

Among the OPS therapists I interviewed, a majority felt that their working conditions impoverished their professional ideals. Carrie, a speech therapist, said, "Certain days, it's just very hard. Staffing-wise, it's a hard trade-off. A few days, you'll have plenty of staff, and most days you won't have enough . . . so short-staffed days mean that you're going to have trouble doing follow-ups and getting things accomplished." She explained that on such days, you end up "not doing everything you are supposed to do in the way you're supposed to."

In addition to bemoaning these "short-staffed days," OPS therapists emphasized how their work required focused personal attention and that it was difficult to "take their time" when patient needs routinely exceeded their allotted time. This led to fast-paced work days, forcing them to prioritize tasks and take shortcuts. For Barry, a physical therapist, "thirty-minute hours" had become a surreal norm, and he felt that time constraints were one of his biggest problems:

> I think a lot of what sort of speeds up time for us [is] not just that we have too many patients assigned to us, but also we have a lot of other factors that play into sort of that ticking clock where we're trying to find the chart, we're trying to find the nurse, we're trying to get a patient who maybe is unavailable because they're probably at x-ray or in the bathroom and so we have to come back.

When this happens, "the patient ends up feeling sort of neglected," which Barry noted was "sort of a strong word," but indicative of the pressures OPS therapists were under.

But, although OPS therapists may have experienced time crunches, their working conditions could be worse. Many days were particularly strenuous because of a high volume of patient referrals for evaluation or therapy. However, OPS therapists did have comparatively more control over when and how they spent their time on the floor than other frontline practitioners such as nurses. For instance, after patients had been evaluated, assessed, and prescribed therapy, OPS therapists were likely to know (or could make an informed guess about) which patients would require future assistance and the number and length of expected therapy sessions. Compared to nurses, some RTs, and most physicians, whose jobs were not referral-based, OPS therapists enjoyed more flexibility in managing their workloads. In short, their position in the health-care labor process allowed them to informally negotiate the unfavorable working conditions that challenged their sense of professionalism and caring ideals.

. . . It Just Got Worse

Of all the practitioners I interviewed, it was nurses with whom I began to *feel* what it's like to work in a factory. Nurses bemoaned the lack of time to perform their work routines adequately and the exacting toll of such fast-paced work. Tim entered nursing to make a difference in people's lives—to "do the right thing, for the right reason." But he wondered if it was possible under the circumstances, and his words were echoed by the majority of nurses I spoke with:

> You don't have enough time to do a good job! You start prioritizing
> off things, and some of the first things to go are patients' hygiene,
> because it's much more important to get the antibiotic in than it
> is to wash the body. It's more important to draw their labs than
> it is to comb their hair. . . . That's really sad. . . . That's when we're
> supposedly appropriately staffed, never mind [on] a short-staffed
> day. . . . It's overwhelming from the get-go: you're frazzled, you
> don't have time for a break, you don't have time to eat, you don't
> have time to go to the bathroom. . . . After a while, *if the nurse
> doesn't get any fuel or any rest, then the nurse starts to break down.*
> I mean, it's a twelve-hour shift—it's not like there's an end close in
> sight. You don't have time to nourish yourself; you end up dehy-
> drated, frazzled, upset, hungry. That situation is just unacceptable.
> It's really, really stressful! (Emphasis added.)

Characterizing a nurse as something resembling an automobile strains the image of professionalism that nursing has so stridently embraced and struggled for. But for Tim and other nurses, the metaphor aptly conveys how they felt during and after a shift: as machines, rather than the idealized professional self. As an oncology nurse explained to me, "we feel like we're constantly going through rapids, you know—just as things calm down, you suddenly get swept into another rapid."

Diane had nursed in Hospital General for over twenty-five years, so by most accounts she was a "survivor." "I don't want to talk bad about doctors," she confided. "They work very hard, but they have their schedules and they can pretty much come and go as they please." Having to be constantly on the floor, Diane feared that staffing problems and the pressure on nurses to get things done jeopardized patient care:

> Sometimes we feel like they [administrators] bombard us with too many patients at once and it is not safe. So a lot of times you are uncomfortable with unsafe conditions. You feel stressed and it is just way too busy! You can't take care of everything when patient levels get really high. It's hard to be and see your coworkers really under stress, but people are trying to do their best and do their job. A lot of times, you feel like you don't have time. It's just too much, [and] overwhelming. It's hard and I think less people are going into the field [nursing] because of this. It is overwhelming mentally and physically, and you have to be organized on top of that. . . . You have to do a lot of multitasking.

For nurses, "getting through the day" meant juggling how to care for patients while also taking care of themselves, a situation that inevitably resulted in them neglecting their own basic needs (i.e., eating, drinking, using the restroom), leading to dissatisfaction and, as one nurse put it, "lots of burn-out."[8] Even though nurse-patient ratios are legally mandated, nurses faced work intensification on a daily basis.[9] Whether they functioned as the "eyes and ears" of physicians or as "thinking nurses," they still took orders not only from physicians but also other groups such as OPS therapists.[10] This compounded the strain of having "to be everywhere and do everything," as nurses were the most frequent presence at the bedside.

For social workers, working conditions ranked highest among their concerns over their professional obligations to patients. Like many of her coworkers, Sheila wondered how she could possibly meet patient needs under the circumstances:

> [The problem is] too many patients and not enough of us. . . . There are people up on the floor that I know could benefit from social work services. But I usually have to really filter it down to the ones that are more critical . . . and that usually means that we see the most extreme cases. . . . So we have to prioritize. I think that the professional ideal or best circumstance would be where you have enough people to help every patient who needs you.

Social workers had been particularly hard hit by understaffing in the hospital. Some had retired or gone on extended sick-leave while others had decided to go part-time or to quit altogether. The department also faced an uphill battle in recruiting and retaining new hires. "The institution keeps expecting more with less," said one social worker, shaking her head in dismay:

> That whole attitude of "OK, there are how many social workers? We can cut down by two or we can cut down by four." . . . "We can just do more with less." . . . That's one of the biggest frustrations for professionals, I think, in a bureaucratic setting like this one: how do you do a good enough job so you can go home feeling like you have accomplished what you want to accomplish despite the fact that maybe there is just not enough time to do everything you want to do?

Social workers thought that the hospital administration was trying to reduce labor costs and increase revenue from patient admissions. In their view, this inevitably led to overwhelming patient ratios, which especially affected them because they were, compared to nurses or physicians, a smaller department, with fewer than fifty full-time employees servicing the entire hospital. Their struggle, as they saw it, highlighted their marginal position as nonmedical ancillary staff in an organizational milieu that prized biomedical knowledge and skills.[11]

For respiratory therapists, things could not get much worse. Expressing the highest level of dissatisfaction with working conditions, RTs thought that inadequate staffing directly compromised their work with any given patient. Like Jason, whom we met at the beginning of this chapter, another senior RT expressed what I heard again and again from others:

> [A main challenge is] having too many patients [and] having too
> high of a workload, which sometimes happens when we're not ade-
> quately staffed. I think, for the most part, staffing has been better
> than in the past, but it's still a problem. But you still find yourself
> always having to triage, because we can't spend the same amount of
> time with every patient, so you have to figure out that. When things
> are like this, you don't apply yourself—you don't use all of your skills
> because you're thinking of what you need to do next.

Compared with physicians and OPS therapists, RTs, like nurses and social workers, were more likely to speak of the constant "triaging"; that is, the daily prioritizing process they engaged in to cope with understaffing, high workloads, and limited time. Consistent with every group other than physicians, RTs lamented the physical and emotional costs of being overworked and its impact on the quality of their care and already fragile occupational status. Their dissatisfaction with working conditions could be because of all the groups, RTs are the least credentialed and thus exercise the least control over their labor. Like the individual nurse, RTs had little say in what physicians ordered as "necessary" respiratory care. However, unlike nurses, who were well represented in the hospital administration and through a strong labor union, RTs lacked any organizational leverage that might improve their working conditions. Ironically, the situation of RTs more closely resembled that of social workers: even though the social workers held postgraduate degrees, they too deployed knowledge that was either devalued or considered "merely" technical.

Patients and Families

Health care requires not only knowledge and technical competence but also interactional skills and a keen ability to "read" people (traditionally seen as "soft skills"), especially given the relationships between practitioners, patients, and their families.[12] These relationships often feature interactions that are often highly emotional or fraught with bad news.[13] Equally significant are the expectations that patients and families bring to the hospital regarding the type of care they should receive.[14] These expectations often go unmet under these conditions and the limits of health-care delivery in the HMO system.[15]

Even though patients are not always "difficult," they are nonetheless ill, in pain, or frequently impatient, given the stress and uncertainty of their hospital stay. Patient distress arises from their perceived lack of control over their situation: being in an unfamiliar setting, feeling handicapped, fearing what may happen to them and what it may mean to their loved ones, feeling unattended, and being confused about how the hospital bureaucracy works are all common experiences of individuals entering total institutions.[16] In turn, it can be challenging for practitioners to care for and get along with patients and families under these circumstances.[17]

My research did not focus on patient attitudes toward practitioners, so I did not formally interview them or seek their views. During my fieldwork, however, I learned that patients and families entered the hospital with a range of preconceptions, including some with lofty expectations of the services they would get (especially if they had never been hospitalized), and some with jaded and cynical attitudes (particularly if they were what practitioners called "frequent flyers," or if they had had a previous negative experience).[18] Practitioners across groups were likely to label certain patients and their families as "needy," "pushy," or "a pain." Typically, this meant that the patient and/or their family demanded more attention than practitioners could or were willing to extend, requested more things than necessary, questioned practitioners' skills, knowledge, and care, or wanted to determine their medical treatment without taking practitioners' recommendations.[19] In short, the relationships and interactions between practitioners, patients, and their families can be stressful if not outright conflictive.

Likewise, the practitioner-patient relationship in Hospital General was further strained by the large proportion of patients who were indigent (many of whom suffered from alcoholism, drug addiction, and/or drug abuse, and came from broken families or the streets), institutionalized (i.e., from nursing homes or jails), and non-English-speaking. According to one administrator, approximately only 25 percent of those receiving care in the hospital were "paying" patients.[20] The socioeconomic gap and cultural differences between practitioners and patients often made it difficult for each to understand (much less trust) the other, even when social workers were present, and in spite of the hospital's translation services in various languages.[21]

Practitioners and patients frequently struggled to establish and maintain the cooperative and trusting relationships necessary for an effective

hospital stay and prompt discharge.[22] This often required delicate negotiation or reparation work by practitioners, who were generally responsible
for strained relationships, which in turn reflected on their reputation and
the hospital's public image. All practitioners shared the view that patients
were to be cared for and satisfied as clients.[23] The occupations, however,
were not held equally responsible for meeting such expectations (especially
by patients and families). These expectations, derived from stereotypes and
patients' experiences, were reinforced by an occupation's status and its role
in the labor process.

It Could Be Worse . . .

A majority of the physicians I interviewed felt that conflicts with patients
and families were a troubling aspect of their work. These conflicts generally resulted from patient noncompliance with treatment, incompatible
personalities, or patients' frustration with what they considered inadequate
quality of care.[24] Dr. Bernstein admitted that conflicts with patients were
common:

> [Sometimes] you're running late and the patient is very upset that
> we were a half hour late, which is not even very late by our stan-
> dards, but you have to try [to understand how they feel]. Sometimes
> you're even late by your standards—you're an hour late or some-
> thing, you know. So if a person is upset with you, your choices are
> to fight back or to let them blow off, and you have to make a choice
> based upon, one, was I right? And two, whether fighting back with
> them is a good thing, you know?

In a similar vein, Dr. Sullivan recalled a particular incident with one of her
patients:

> Sometimes you can't avoid having conflicts with patients. For
> example, I remember there was this patient that was totally
> bummed that she had a life-threatening condition and she had
> totally bonded with the nurses and they were like friends. She saw
> me as the "mean" doctor who is insisting on this or that because
> I thought it was good for her medical health. It ended up in a big
> conflict. . . . And I basically lost her ability to help me with what I

> thought was medically good for her . . . because we would not see
> eye to eye and not all the things that she wanted were necessarily
> in her best interest.

Though physicians had unpleasant encounters with patients, these remained more a nuisance than a chronic problem, because compared with other practitioners, they spent the least amount of time at the bedside. Their visibility (or invisibility) is telling; physicians can exert authority from a distance and avoid direct face-to-face conflict with those they treat. Likewise, physicians believed that they approached patient relationships in purely medical terms, or with what has been termed "detached concern."[25] Consequently, they could afford patients not "liking them," thinking of them as "emotionally unattached," or not seeing "eye to eye" with them. Physicians may have encountered unruly or uncooperative patients and families, but "the white coat" evoked a different set of rules regarding their relationship and interactions with them.

. . . It Just Got Worse

As with working conditions, all the other groups voiced significantly more concern over problems with patients and families. It was not surprising to find that an overwhelming majority of RTs viewed conflicts with patients and families as a daily hurdle, given their relatively low status in the hospital hierarchy and their regular presence at the bedside. For many, it was "not easy to get along with patients." As she reflected on difficult patients, a senior RT shared her frustration:

> I've had patients tell me, "Well, I don't like you." I'm a pretty crusty
> old woman and I tell them, "I'm not here for you to like me, I'm here
> to help you get better and get the hell outta here!" And they usu-
> ally go, "Oh, okay." And I say, "So do you want your treatment now
> or not?" Then you have the patients who just get mean. . . . I don't
> think they realize, "Okay, these people [RTs] are here to take care of
> me and help me get better, but I'm going to bite their head off and
> make their life a living hell the whole time I'm here." I tell them, "I'll
> be honest with you, you're not really helping yourself. . . . Pissing off
> everybody who tries to take care of you does not help."

Respiratory therapists had developed thick skins because of patients who disliked, dismissed, or simply disrespected them as merely workers instead of esteemed professionals. Tom recalled a troublesome patient who "was just a slug. I mean, just, grrrr! He wanted us to do everything but he didn't do anything to help himself and he was just rude to every RT." The rudeness eventually became too much to bear: "This guy really got to me, and I finally went, 'Oh, I'm going to tell this guy . . . ' And I just told him what an asshole he was, you know. I said, 'Listen, I'm coming in here to help you and you're being a total prick about this and I don't appreciate you being an asshole.'" Tom left the room, informed the nurse what had happened, and walked away. The patient complained to all the other practitioners, who "just blew it off." Summarizing the incident, Tom said, "I just told him the truth, hoping that maybe he wakes up and he'd be a little bit more appropriate."

While few RTs would likely endorse what some might consider un-professional vernacular, they commonly recalled instances when a patient simply "got to them." Most RTs reported trying hard to repair the patient-practitioner relationship after these awkward interactions; the repair work summoned conflict-defusing skills and coping strategies, but still left their professional self on the ropes.[26]

Surprisingly, despite significant differences in status and levels of exper-tise, OPS therapists similarly viewed conflicts with patients and families as compromising their professionalism and ability to care. "There is always a patient who wants too much of you," Bill said. Such patients are "dealing with too many other things—again, social problems, emotional and mental illness, or addiction—that prevent them from being able to really partici-pate in their care." He added that these patients "can be a problem—a bur-den, even. It makes it very hard to work with them because they tend to be belligerent, very frustrated, and they are just not nice: they insult you and don't treat you as a professional . . . when you're trying to do your job."

Good relationships with patients and their families were critical to OPS therapists, as their jobs required frequent one-on-one contact at the bed-side. All the OPS therapists agreed that the relationship necessary for ade-quate care could be seriously jeopardized when patient and practitioner expectations or personalities clashed. Pointing to this, Julie, a speech thera-pist, spoke of a patient and his family:

> I have a patient right now that does not want any of my services,
> and he is not listening to any of my recommendations. So what am I
> going to do for him? What kind of therapy is that? It is not therapy.
> It is forcing something on him that he doesn't want, so I discharged
> him. I said, "Fine, if that is what you want." It's hard to deal with
> patients like that day in and day out. . . . And the family—I think you
> need a good family to work with that respects you as a professional.
> It is harder to do therapy with somebody when a family is frustrated
> or unsupportive, or thinks you don't know what you are doing.

Given their frequent and personal contact with patients, conflicts were more likely for OPS therapists, and this aligns them with the other occupational groups that were present at the bedside more regularly. This visibility heightened patient and family expectations, which in turn compromised the professional respect sought by OPS therapists. Though they considered themselves closer to physicians than other health practitioners, their rehabilitative work inevitably involved physically painful and psychologically stressful interactions with patients they could not evade, unlike physicians.

An overwhelming majority of social workers reported having similarly strained encounters with patients on a daily basis. In general, social workers attributed these conflicts to stereotypes of them as "welfare assistants" or "secretaries to the poor." Yet some of these perceptions ring true, as social workers often dealt with indigent patients who were familiar with social services outside the hospital.[27] As one social worker explained:

> A lot of times, they [patients] expect things that you are not there
> for. . . . I'm like, "No, that's your job, that's not my job to find you a
> doctor when you leave the hospital. . . ." Then they ask you, "Would
> you take me there?" I tell them, "I can give you the phone book, you
> can find a doctor, and you can call a taxi," and that's what I'd have to
> do. . . . Because this is what the patient or family can do: "Here's the
> phone book. These are the doctors. You need to call them and ask
> them if they can accept a medical patient right now."

Frequently, social workers said that patients wanted them to perform menial tasks, rejecting their counseling support and dismissing their knowledge about the health-care system. I routinely observed how these patient-family expectations annoyed social workers and reinforced their perception of being devalued in the hospital. And more than any other group, social workers spoke of the emotional and physical toll of potential incendiary interactions. As Bernard, an experienced social worker, explained:

> We [social workers] can face very hostile patients or violent situations sometimes and we have to do some stress processing afterwards. . . . Down the road, it could have the flavor of a post-traumatic episode for us because all of a sudden you become very alert and very aware of somebody who reminds you of that patient or family and the whole incident. You just get kind of scared, because you know what could or what did happen. A few of us have been physically assaulted. . . . We have sometimes called hospital security. Sometimes I have security stand by out of the way so that the family doesn't see it, in case they get volatile or violent. If I have misjudged them, I in no way want to insult them by having the police there.

Bernard added, "I have had conflicts with patients that have been combative; we try different things to defuse their anger or frustration, but sometimes the only way to resolve it is by calling law enforcement, our own hospital police, to assist."

In this respect, social workers resembled OPS therapists, because the visibility of their interventions (whether biomedical or psychological in nature) often strained interactions with patients and families. Ironically, their nonmedical role (i.e., showing up sans the white coat or medical scrubs) was occasionally an advantage, as social workers often interacted with patients in a more egalitarian manner to avoid conflict or to accomplish their treatment goals.

For all the nurses I interviewed, patient and family conflicts inflicted personal insult, great stress, frustration, dissatisfaction, and burnout. Typically, nurses reported facing patients who treated them as handmaidens and unskilled workers. Faye had worked in pediatrics for many years, and her experience is illustrative:

> No matter what drink I brought her, she wanted something else. So I'd go to get apple juice; meanwhile, her pills would disappear. At first, I thought she'd taken them, but usually it would always take her fifteen to twenty minutes to take the pills. That day, suddenly

not only were they gone, but so were all the wrappers. The wrappers were in the trash; she had been tricking me all the time. . . . Also, she would always throw the wrappers and stuff on her bed sheet or on the floor, expecting me to pick up after her, and I would tell her, "I'm not your maid, clean them up." She thought I would never realize what she was doing, and she thought I was there to clean up after her.

It is not surprising that nurses experienced more conflicts with patients and families because, of all the groups, they spent the most time at the bedside. Besides contending with degrading stereotypes, nurses faced patient and family expectations that they viewed as unrealistic and/or unacceptably demeaning of them as professionals. As one nurse working in an adult unit explained:

Oh, they [patients and families] have still the stereotype of the nurses in a starched white uniform and caps and going about caring for the patient, holding their hand, bathing them, and giving a massage every day. The nurse is a handmaiden for the doctor. All those Florence Nightingale stereotypes continue to this day, so that is a problem. . . . And then you have the patients that are cranky and rude and the family that is constantly nagging at you for this little thing or the other 'cause they think you are not doing a good job. . . . You know, I've been "fired" by patients before, because they say they don't like you. All of us [nurses] have had that at some point. . . . It's kind of par for the course as a nurse to have conflicts like that with patients. . . . It can get tiresome and it really can lower your morale as a professional.

In general, nurses felt that their authority on the floor was commonly and openly questioned by patients and families (which only fueled their discontent with the occupational hierarchy). Further, when a nurse-patient relationship went awry, the nurse had to repair it, as the event might tarnish their reputation on the floor, and they could not as easily avoid the bedside as a practitioner from another group. It was nurses who absorbed the anxiety and demands of the ill and infirm; more than any other group, they had to balance satisfying what they considered petty requests by patients and defending their professional self.

While all the occupational groups were "under the gun" in this regard, the barrel seemed to point directly at some of them. Their authority in the hospital, public perceptions and misperceptions about their occupation, the degree of bedside visibility, and the frequency and nature of patient contact all shaped the interactions practitioners had with patients and families.[28]

Material Resources

Resources such as money, physical space and facilities, the availability of equipment, supplies, and medical technology are finite, and their scarcity can potentially foster conflict and compromise patient care.[29] As in any complex organization, many formal and informal negotiations influence how these resources are distributed and managed in the hospital.[30] Although there were marked differences in the proportion of practitioners that emphasized working conditions and practitioner-patient relationships, this was not the case regarding material resources. Rather, the number of practitioners who identified material resources as a challenge was smaller and very similar across the groups (less than half for all the groups except nurses, where slightly over half voiced concerns).

While it is difficult to confirm the veracity of claims about limited resources without detailed information, I was able to find some crude estimates about the hospital's revenues and expenditures. These data are limited (i.e., they do not provide occupational breakdowns), but they still provide a base context for considering practitioners' claims about resource scarcity. For example, based on official financial report data, Hospital General was in some ways better off than two comparable hospitals in the area, with higher gross patient revenues and significantly higher tax deductions and exemptions.[31] Likewise, it reported having significantly higher charity contributions and donations. Considering its total operating expenses, as well as specific items such as salaries and wages, Hospital General appeared to have financial and material resources less available to other institutions. This advantage, however, was not always reflected in practitioners' perceptions; they did not unanimously believe that things were better in Hospital General than in other comparable private or for-profit institutions.

While physicians arguably exercised more influence than other practitioners in how monies were allocated and used, some of them still felt deprived, at least relatively. "The performance of my job, of my professional skills, is constrained by limited high tech," Dr. Lancaster explained. "It is constantly exhausting trying to make sure that there is a machine to do the test for the patient who needs it. . . . And it makes our work so much more difficult, and our ability to practice as we would like to do it is sometimes on the line because of this." Other physicians voiced similar concerns, but the fact is that Hospital General spent more dollars on medical equipment than two other area hospitals. Likewise, in a national survey assessing over five thousand institutions in 2005, the hospital ranked among the highest for "key technology-related services and availability," which are considered crucial resources for physicians' diagnosis and treatment. It is likely that while physicians at Hospital General may experience some shortage of equipment, physicians in similar institutions could have it worse.

Unlike physicians, who focused primarily on high technology, RTs, OPS therapists, and nurses commonly spoke of lacking specific medications, adequate facilities, therapy supplies, and basic equipment. Bryan, a young RT, said that "there are always problems related to resources"—problems that frequently translated into perceptions of professional malfeasance:

> For us [RTs], most of the time, it's a matter of what meds we can use for patients. There are some drugs that are very expensive and the hospital won't allow us to use them. For example, Zolfanex is one, where we might be able to help the patient, but we can't use it because of the cost, and that is a big issue, because you can't do your work as you should and then patients and others think it's because you are not making the right calls or [don't] have the knowledge and skills to be on top of what's best for patients.

Nurses also claimed to get "the short end of the stick" when it came to resources. Bertha, a nurse in an adult medical-surgical unit, complained about an older part of the unit: "Less space, really cramped, and much more dirty." A pediatric nurse concurred about the lack of resources:

> It is so much easier when you have everything at your fingertips. If I could have a blood pressure machine and a pill pack with heart monitors and everything in every single room, it would make my day a million times easier, rather than searching around the floor trying to find that one blood pressure machine to do a blood

pressure on a kid or a pulse ox. . . . We only have two showers for thirty-two patients! But definitely not having the tools can be a problem . . . and then you start wondering if other professionals have to go through this kind of stuff.

Again, it was difficult to verify these concerns based on other data, but a rough examination of hospital expenditures showed that during the period of this study, Hospital General spent more funds on supplies and more money on buildings and renovations than the two other area institutions. Moreover, the hospital was expanding and had recently embarked on a massive construction project to upgrade key facilities. Yet I often observed nurses in the predicament of not having something they needed (e.g., missing the right bandage, or having to wait to use a blood pressure machine), and I certainly saw the need for physical renovation of some older sections of the hospital. However, if resource scarcity hindered practitioners, it was in terms of their reaching an even higher level of service than patients already received, and the hospital seemed to be investing significantly in renovations and new construction.

It is also likely that practitioners had become good at making do with what they had. For example, Dilan, a speech therapist, spoke of having to personally "come up" with materials he deemed necessary for his patients:

> I am pretty good about materials, given that we don't have a lot of resources and many times we don't have what we need at all. You have to get creative with the materials that you have to make it work, or bring your own stuff. . . . There are all kinds of new things we could be doing that we know about because of cutting-edge research, but we can't perform at that level because you don't have what you need.

As was the case with other groups, some OPS therapists saw minimal resources as undermining patient care by restricting what their professional training enabled them to do. Social workers were no different. "It's been a rough year just because of some big changes in funding to our department," a senior social worker said. "The hospital was funding social workers, but it severely cut back on some adult services and pediatrics for coverage of social services. . . . And I don't think it's in the best interest of patient care." For social workers it was funding, rather than equipment or supplies per se, that was crucial to being able to fulfill their professional promise. Even without other data, one can be fairly confident that as the lowest group on the health-care totem pole, social workers operated on a shoestring budget.

Who Is To Blame?

Given how the occupational hierarchy and division of labor in the hospital structure the collective interests of each of these groups, one might reasonably expect them to hold each other responsible for their misfortune. But if we expand our view of the hospital labor force beyond these practitioners to the hospital administration, it is hardly surprising that physicians, nurses, RTs, OPS therapists, and social workers alike pointed their collective finger at these higher circles of power. Indeed, collective resentment was hierarchical rather than lateral, as I seldom heard one group blame another for soaking up resources unjustly. Yet, again and again, the hospital administration was targeted, not only for lack of resources, but also for troubling working conditions. As a physician put it:

> The administration says, "No, you are not making enough money to get this extra machine, so we are not going to give it to you." The administration looks at the bottom line. If this were a physician or somebody who worked closely with us making this decision, they would say, "Oh, absolutely, let's get the machine! There's no reason why three times a day you should roll the $300,000 digital acquisition system into a van and drive it down the street so that we can provide care."

A nurse shared his frustration:

> The administration and the politics within the hospital affects what we get and the equipment you have. . . . Sometimes it is hard for us to do our jobs as well as we would like because the administration says this or that. . . . Sometimes I wish we would have given them [patients] another day or a certain piece of equipment; that would make our job just much easier, but we can't seem to get it because of the funding—because of the administration and the politics they play. . . . That probably is the most frustrating. But I try to look past it and not even think about it, and just go with

what I have. But when it comes up and it is a major issue, it is very frustrating.

The majority of physicians and nurses I spoke with viewed the administration as always chasing the "bottom line"; that is, engaging in cost-cutting and profit-making at the expense of quality patient care and the practitioners' professional reputations. OPS therapists expressed similar sentiments. For example, a physical therapist pondered how often she lacked necessary materials to perform her work: "I understand that some equipment and supplies can be expensive, but sometimes they are not. . . . It's politics, you know. It's mostly the administration that is a problem. We need the resources and they [administrators] do not see it the same way we do because . . . to the administration is about the money. . . . They don't see what we see or what we go through when we're with the patient."

Respiratory therapists were also quick to blame the "higher-ups." As one RT adamantly told me:

> Well, it's pretty pathetic. . . . The CEO takes a nice bonus of
> $300,000 and we have to be chasing the equipment down the hall or
> we can't use this medication or that medication because it's a little
> more costly. . . . Some days we even have to rent ventilators because
> we don't have enough of them, but the administration decides to
> spend money on new chairs for their office. . . . They [administra-
> tors] are not the ones on the floor, and they only think of the bottom
> line, you know.

Although most social workers agreed that the administration had slightly "changed its tune" in the last few years by looking at social services in a more favorable light, they also thought circumstances were far from ideal. As Sarah, who had practiced in the hospital for two decades, explained:

> I think that the administration holds so much power. Frequently,
> they [administrators] look at budget or look at programs from the
> perspective of "do they make us any money" rather than from the
> perspective of "we are a teaching/training hospital and we have
> a mission. . . ." We [social workers] do not bring money into the
> hospital, we don't turn [a] profit for the hospital, and they [admin-

istrators] think of us as a "cost." . . . I think that's always been a real
conflict between the administration and the services like us.

What struck me over time as I listened to these concerns is how distinct they were from any critique that each group might level against one
another. As the quotes above attest, practitioners saw administrative "politics" as the source of most problems, with the administration holding too
much power and with the "bottom line" and "profit" coming before patient
care and professional integrity. And while these criticisms may be valid,
it is also interesting that practitioners rarely if ever saw disputes between
themselves as a matter of "politics," though they clearly were. It is here that
professional ideology legitimates the position of practitioners in relation
to hospital administration and reinforces their occupational status. For the
professional, politics cuts against their faith in science, their sense of objectivity, and their calling to serve others. As the physician above argued,
the administration uses the bottom line to deny requests that his colleagues
would consider absolutely reasonable; it is a shame when the bottom line
endangers a patient or hinders one's medical practice.

This antagonism between professionals and state or corporate power
has a history as long as the existence of professional groups.[32] The professional has always claimed an allegiance to a "greater good" than either crass
power or profit, both of which might compromise their disinterested pursuit of, in the case of medicine and health care, healing and the well-being
of patients. But it is striking—and this is its ideological appeal, of course—
how the critique of administration politics (valid as it may be) masks the
power relations and politics among groups of practitioners themselves.
And to the degree that practitioners have little or no voice in how funding decisions are made and resources allocated, their critique resonates
with a professional ethos of egalitarian participation that is being ignored
if not mocked by administrative fiat. Consequently, the critique serves to
"circle the wagons" by bonding practitioners to one another and against
the hospital administration. Again, none of this impugns practitioners or
their criticism of administrative politics, for this is a function of ideological
claims: they direct attention, inform opinion, and identify "culprits." But if
the ideological halo of Hospital General is "teamwork," then its antithesis
in the minds of practitioners is "administration politics."

At the end of the day, diverse interoccupational interests can converge in the name of professionalism against a separate class of managers en-sconced in the hospital bureaucracy.[33] The practitioner view that some may get more than others at certain times is ultimately balanced by a (not necessarily accurate) consensus that everyone is in the same boat vis-à-vis hospital administrators and the forces pushing to maximize hospital prof-its. Ironically, this unified outlook may blur occupation status distinctions and yet still impede any collective mobilization on behalf of organizational changes that might enhance professional collaboration.[34] Other than nurses acting through their union, no other group has been interested or able to effectively mobilize any significant challenge to administration policies or directives that they deem unjust or unfair.

The fact that less than half of the practitioners considered material re-sources a serious problem raises another issue. When thinking about un-derstaffing, time constraints, and heavy workloads as "resource" issues, one could argue that the most serious problems in Hospital General *are social in nature*, be they working conditions or patient/family conflicts. When we view these "people problems" as requiring social rather than material solutions, a key point emerges: for professional workers, social relations embody more risk, hold more meaning, and bestow more benefits than materials resources such as technology, supplies, or space. If Andrew Abbott is correct regarding professionalism, which he says is primarily characterized by jurisdictional disputes between occupations, then my in-terviews confirm the social context of these disputes in the organizational setting of the hospital. It is not necessarily control over technology that matters in professional work; rather, it is the management of relationships, whether of clients or other professional groups, that tips the scales. In this case, it is necessary to explore how these groups manage these challenges (read: social relationships) on a daily basis. What strategies do different groups deploy to handle and cope with these problems, and how are pro-fessionalism and caring implicated through these strategies? It is to these questions that I now turn.

Chapter 6

Crossing the Line

Sometimes you just have to do what it takes to move things along.
—PHYSICAL THERAPIST

ET BACK in an old wing of the hospital, the neurology unit was a messy place, with narrow hallways and small rooms, limited workspace for staff, and what seemed like a closet-sized break room for nurses. One day, I stuck close to Ruth, the shift charge nurse; in addition to her managerial duties, she had three patients to assist, because the unit was understaffed. Ruth was a veteran with over thirty years of nursing practice, and she had spent about twenty-five years working in Hospital General. She knew everyone and everything and everyone knew her.

She had taken over one of the "bad" assignments, caring for a belligerent female patient who had been found unconscious on the street and was being evaluated by two residents from the neurology service, whom the nurses referred to as Tommy and Chris. As Ruth and I entered this patient's room, the patient started yelling uncontrollably, growling, spitting, kicking, and threatening to pull her IV off and leave. She simply did not want me there, and Ruth told me, "It's best if you don't come in."

I quickly exited the room, and as I walked past Tommy, he said, "Don't worry, she doesn't like anybody right now. . . . We think she might have a brain tumor."

Ruth returned from the room and asked the residents whether they had the brain scan results. Finding that the imaging results had been posted, the residents and Ruth huddled around the computer, looking at the colorful pictures and discussing what they saw. The residents thought the patient had a tumor that required surgery. "You see this here?" Chris said. "I think that is the tumor."

"Well, it is not so clear," Ruth cautioned. "It could be, but it does not mean it is malignant."

Ruth's beeper beckoned us to another patient. After I helped her change the bed, move the patient, and prepare him for lunch, we returned to the station and found it in complete chaos. The female patient had attempted to leave the floor after Tommy and Chris had told her she would need brain surgery because she had a tumor. They managed to get her back in her room, and Ruth settled her down. She promised to call the patient's brother, as the woman had requested.

After leaving the patient, Ruth confronted the residents, angrily asking them why they had told the patient she needed brain surgery. Looking at each other, they replied, "Because she has a brain tumor."

"No, you *think* she has a tumor," Ruth retorted, "and *you* think she has to have surgery. But we are not certain of that. . . . I've been around a long time and I know that sometimes you guys are wrong or the scans are wrong."

Chris insisted that without surgery the patient could die. Ruth abruptly ended the exchange by scolding them about their bad judgment. "You better make sure to talk to your attending," Ruth stated. "Otherwise, I will."

The patient's brother arrived a few hours later and spoke with Chris, the only resident on the floor at the time. Chris told the visibly concerned man that his sister had a brain tumor that needed surgery. The man asked if the doctors were certain about the need for an operation. "She doesn't want the surgery," he added, to which Chris responded, "We know that's what she has, and you have to make her understand that she has to have the surgery."

After Chris left, however, Ruth approached the patient's brother and said, "You know, I don't think it is clear she has a brain tumor and, by the way, she doesn't have to have the surgery if she doesn't want to." The man seemed confused, and his concern grew as Ruth continued: "I've worked on this floor with this type of patient for a long time and I can tell you that even if that's what she has, surgery may not be the best thing. . . . Sometimes they don't recover well and they are worse off than they were. It's up to her."

Things went from bad to worse when the brother told Ruth that his sister wanted to be discharged: "They [the physicians] can't make her stay, right?" The residents stood outside the room, trying to persuade the man to have his sister stay for the surgery, but she had made up her mind. Ruth removed her IV; the patient got dressed and left within the hour.

As the residents left, Ruth cast a parting shot: "You can't make patients do what you want, even if you are right." It was around 3:30 in the afternoon; there were still another three and a half hours left in the shift, and I could not wait to go home. By the looks on everyone's faces, neither could they.

Ruth challenged the physicians by insisting that their diagnosis was premature. While she did this informally, it was clear that she was ready to move up the chain of command and contact the attending in charge. During my observations at Hospital General, I noticed countless instances of breached professional boundaries that rarely evoked any lasting concerns. While the physicians above insisted that they had the correct diagnosis, they never told Ruth that she had no right to pass judgment on their medical opinion (perhaps because they were residents). Instead, Ruth's transgression was considered reasonable, because she had many years of intimate experience with neurology patients and because nurses and physicians share an understanding that diagnoses can be inaccurate or incorrect altogether.

Boundary work of this type opens a window into how the professional self negotiates the hospital status hierarchy as one carefully evaluates the potential for more serious conflicts. Similar forms of boundary work not only reinforce status rankings in Hospital General, but they are also critical in uniting the professional self with the caring ideals I discussed earlier. The seemingly fluid integration of all these groups in providing health care requires that practitioners find common ground in an ideology of caring despite working conditions that confront, confound, and compromise it. Although it is based on practitioners striving to provide emotive caring, boundary work *reinforces the very occupational hierarchy that undermines this normative ideal.* As this process reproduces the occupational roles and exclusiveness I have explored up to now, it also imbues the professional self with the caring ideals to which all practitioners aspire and struggle to live up to.[1] In other words, practitioners cross occupational boundaries to "get things done," and this is ultimately justified and symbolically supported by their desire to care for, as much as about, their patients. That practitioners disagreed over the issue at hand, as we shall see, did not impugn their caring but was a declaration of it. This process is more contingent than previously outlined by macrostructural accounts, and by analyzing how boundary work reinforces a sense of occupational membership and distinction at the micro (bedside) level, I am able to shed light on how the structure of professional work and the caring ideology are reproduced at the macro (organizational) level.

Boundary Work in Health Care

The concept of boundaries has been extensively developed in research on ethnicity and race, gender and sexuality, class, and the professions and work.[2] Cynthia Fuchs Epstein provides a useful definition of boundaries as marking "the social territories of human relations, signaling who ought to be admitted and who excluded. Moreover, there are rules that guide and regulate traffic, and these rules instruct on the conditions under which boundaries may be crossed."[3] In the case of health-care workers, the organizational hierarchy and authority relations of the hospital are constantly being traversed by various occupational groups during patient care. Perhaps no other work setting provides as many occasions of such interdependency of distinct professional groups, whether sequentially (for chronic conditions) or at a given point in time (for emergency room or acute care). Areas of medical specialization often constitute clear boundaries among practitioners of similar authority and power (e.g., brain vs. heart surgery, oncology vs. orthopedics), but I focus on where *hierarchical professional roles* were separated primarily through symbolic distinctions between "curing" and "caring," "skilled" and "unskilled," and "diagnostic" and "technical" labor. It is these occupational boundaries that were regularly crossed, and I show how the status hierarchy is reproduced through practitioner interaction at the point of health-care provision.[4]

Eliot Freidson, in particular, has argued that medicine's successful boundary demarcation, expansion of professional jurisdiction, and autonomous practice are part of a larger process of social domination.[5] This structural-level observation has been empirically supported by microlevel analyses of boundary work in various health-care contexts.[6] What these studies underscore is how professional cohesion and distinction are reproduced, and so too the occupational status hierarchy emphasized by most structural accounts. Yet another body of microlevel research posits how boundary work among health professionals indicates more contingent power dynamics whereby groups traditionally viewed as subordinate often exercise a fair degree of influence over matters such as diagnosis, patient care, and the role of dominant practitioners.[7] Despite how such fine-grained microanalyses portend meaningful and lasting changes among professional status groups (a scenario I will return to later), these important studies of social reproduction via boundary work still portray an occupational hierarchy that is stubbornly intact. And while many health-care practitioners are shown to have usurped the exclusive rights of physicians to diagnose and treat patients, they have yet to fundamentally alter the *knowledge criteria or ideological preferences* that characterize practitioner status hierarchies.

I too found that boundary work reinforces practitioner cohesion and distinction at the organizational level, but I also argue that such boundary work upholds an ideology of caring that obscures how the occupational hierarchy undermines caring. Specifically, crossing boundaries reinforces practitioners' ideological commitment to caring while masking how the emotional work and "soft skills" associated with emotive caring have been rendered secondary to the esoteric knowledge and technical skills considered central to biomedical diagnosis and intervention. A consistent finding of microlevel studies of health-care boundary work is how subordinate groups appropriate the discourse of biomedical science in their struggles (whether successful or not) with other practitioners. What is overlooked, in my view, is how these struggles all operate within a hegemonic discourse of attaining and deploying codified esoteric knowledge; that is, a discourse that reinforces an occupational hierarchy based more on formal education and credentialing than the tacit, experiential knowledge derived from systematic, intimate, and often time-consuming interactions with patients.[8]

Boundary Work on the Hospital Floor

Boundary work became evident not only during my observations on the floor but also through interviews with all five occupational groups. In general, all the practitioners reported that others crossed into what they considered their own occupational jurisdictions. On the floor, these crossings constituted three types of boundary work. *Performing another's "nonmedical" tasks* involves practitioners doing a variety of less skilled or unskilled tasks, such as feeding, changing, or moving a patient, or taking a phone order. *Transgressing the diagnostic line* involves questioning another's knowledge, providing a diagnosis in lieu of an existing one, proposing possible treatments, and claiming knowledge over biomedical issues outside the typical purview of one's training. *Dismissing others' recommendations* involves ignoring another's recommendations, specifications, and/or requests for work or treatment. It is important to note that practitioners engaged in boundary work with a tacit understanding that this was acceptable as long as it was *reasonable*, based on "do no harm" expectations regarding patient well-being, in situ evaluations of who would prevail in any given set of negotiations, and the potential costs should the transgression be pursued further (such as formal disciplinary action by management).

Performing Another's "Nonmedical" Tasks

A phone conversation between a nurse and a physician in an adult medical-surgical unit illustrates the negotiations over performing others' tasks. During her demanding routine, which she generally faced with a dry sense of humor, Valerie expressed to me several times that she was "tired of doing [the physician's] job for him" when he needed to order new drug prescriptions for his patients because of some unforeseen reaction or change of events.

Toward the end of her shift, Valerie answered a phone call from the physician, who asked her to take his order because he was too busy with other patients to make it to her floor. Valerie explained that he needed to come write the new order himself in the patient's chart; that was protocol.

From the tone of her voice and her demeanor, I could tell that Valerie was clearly frustrated as the physician insisted that she take a "verbal order" over the phone. "That is not my job," she replied. "It is your job to come here and write the order in the chart." Legal regulations stipulate that only physicians can order medications, and if Valerie were to take a verbal order and something went wrong, she could be sanctioned. Even so, Valerie eventually agreed to write in the physician's order, warning him that this was "the last time" she would do such a thing.

"Sure, he thinks I'm sitting here picking my nose," she said sardonically, hanging up the phone. "I have six patients to take care of, and I have to do his job too?"

Valerie's interaction with the physician underscores how boundaries separating occupational groups could be temporarily crossed. In this and many other cases I observed, taking a physician's verbal order was considered a task that did not require a specialized set of skills. That Valerie wrote in the order as if she were the physician never led anyone to doubt who was officially supposed to do what. Still, this example also illustrates how low-level conflict frequently pervaded practitioner interactions. As other studies have shown, interoccupational struggles often take the form of overt conflict on the floor.[9] The nurse justified the crossing in terms of the patient's well-being and not because a superior asked her. This type of boundary work led to conflicts that were "chronic" among occupational groups. Pointing to this issue, a physical therapist explained:

> Sometimes, because of things on the floor, there is a little bit of
> misunderstanding about their [nurses'] roles. I know there's a big
> issue about it. I think our department is working on . . . whose role
> is what. Like, there are certain expectations the nurses have of the
> physical therapists, and certain expectations the therapists have
> of the nurses. Sometimes they don't jive and then it causes some
> conflict. . . . They ask you to do routine things that are part of what
> they have to do.

Although most of this boundary work did not result in full, blown-out confrontations, sometimes it remained unresolved, and a group might take formal action by pursuing the issue up the hospital hierarchy. The following account by a social worker, speaking of organ transplant denials, is representative of this:

> What happens in those cases is that the physician goes to the family
> and says, "The committee met and because of these reasons, she
> [the patient] is not a candidate." Lousy job, but this particular physi-
> cian wanted the social worker to come to the family conference
> and explain what the psychosocial evaluation showed that made
> her not a candidate. It was at that point that we had to say, "That is
> not our role," and we had to talk to the medical director so that he
> could resolve the issue. Luckily, the medical director talked with his
> colleague and said, "That is not their [social workers'] role . . . and
> it is our job as a physician, a lousy job, to go to them and say, "I'm
> sorry." There are those times when your [professional] boundaries
> are sort of pressed. I think it is easier for us [the social workers on

the transplant team], but in other parts of the hospital that is not the case at all.

Occupational boundaries were "pressed"—reinterpreted and assigned new meaning—given the shifting conditions under which practitioners worked. In practice, occupational boundaries were open to interpretation, and boundary crossings reflected a collective strategy to make things work on the hospital floor. Practitioners had to weigh what was expected of them and what they could actually do—two very different things when circumstances appeared unmanageable or when others seemed unavailable to lighten the load or "put out the fire."

Performing another's "nonmedical" tasks also occurred because of misguided expectations about the distinct roles occupational groups played under difficult working conditions.[10] As I followed a nurse in the ENT (ear, nose, and throat) unit, it became apparent that she had too many patients and was playing catch-up. As Nancy told me, she was "just trying to survive the day." She had five patients with limited mobility who required assistance for the most basic everyday life activities. Several times during the morning, one patient or another asked Nancy to help them move, sit up, get out of bed, go to the bathroom, or eat, and she started rushing to provide medications on time. Nancy managed to fulfill most of these requests during the morning, but as the afternoon arrived, she had fallen behind in her paperwork and charting.

While removing medications from the drug-dispensing machine at the nurses' station, she saw Laura, one of the occupational therapists, walking toward the main floor exit. Nancy asked Laura if she could move one of Nancy's patients for her. Laura hesitated and said that she was running late for a patient evaluation because they were short-staffed, and she clarified to Nancy that she was there to do therapy only. After Nancy pleaded that she was "swamped" and would really appreciate her helping this one time, Laura went in the patient's room by herself, moved the patient, and hastily left the floor.

At the heart of Nancy's request and Laura's compliance was a shared experience of being overworked with too many patients and a shared understanding of the unthreatening nature of the request. Likewise, Nancy and Laura tacitly agreed that not moving the patient could result in a "big headache," such as the patient launching a formal complaint to an administrator, or in some other problem, such as the patient developing a bedsore. Performing what are considered another's "nonmedical" tasks becomes reasonable not only when practitioners determine that cooperation benefits interoccupational relations (i.e., "I'm doing you a favor and maybe you'll do me a favor when I need it") but also when the symbolic boundary markers, in this case between skilled and unskilled work, were not being challenged.

Early in my research, I was on another adult medical-surgical floor, shadowing Linda, a nurse who regularly cared for five patients. Linda seemed tired and frazzled as she ran around the floor with what seemed like an endless list of tasks. One of her patients was a homeless, young African American male who had been admitted through the emergency room with an acute oral abscess. As we walked toward his room, Linda told me about how unfortunate it was that this "very pleasant, good guy" was homeless. Upon entering the room, Linda asked him if he wanted to see a social worker. "Maybe they [social services] can help you sort things out a little bit," she said reassuringly. Lying on his side, he avoided making eye contact with me as Linda checked his IV and looked at his mouth. After leaving the room, Linda immediately phoned in a request for a social worker.

As the day went by, there was no sign of the social worker. Linda learned that this was not a priority case and that Social Services was overwhelmed with other referrals. During our late lunch in the nurses' break room, Linda spoke about having "to do some talking" with the patient because he needed it. "You know, it's not my job. . . . That is what they [social workers] are here for, because we [nurses] have a lot of other things to do." Linda remarked how frequently nurses have to "put out fires" by doing someone else's job. "We can't let things go undone. We can't say no to the patient," she said, deeply frustrated. "We're there and they see us, but they [other services] can always say, 'I'm sorry, we can't get there today.'"

After lunch, the social worker had still not arrived, so Linda hatched a plan. She made sure everyone got their medications, cleaned up a couple of wounds, made her most urgent calls, and tried to tie up loose ends so that she would have some time to talk to "the depressed guy." When we finally got to his room, Linda said that she did not know when Social Services would be able to see him, but she would be happy to talk if he wanted. He nodded as I left the room, and Linda stayed with him for about forty-five minutes. Afterwards, Linda and I spoke, and she explained how she had

had to improvise some psychotherapy, even though she was not an "expert." Once again, with a heavy sigh, she told me that it was not her job, but it had to be done for the patient's well-being.

I routinely observed similar instances of how work boundaries (skilled vs. unskilled) between different occupational groups were momentarily blurred (yet reaffirmed) so that the provision of care could proceed with only temporary disruptions. For example, Jill spoke of how physical therapists often did nurses' work without it becoming a big problem:

> If we [physical therapists] do work with them [nurses], sometimes it's negotiating whose job is what, and what really is our purpose. It's not a big deal, but sometimes I feel like nurses don't understand that our services have to be there: we have to be progressing a patient; it needs to be towards a specific goal, like going home; and it needs to be therapeutic in the sense that we're teaching, we're letting the patient do as much as they can for themselves. Sometimes nurses want us to come in there and get their patient up or they want us to help pull—they want our muscle strength to help pull them or move them around in bed or whatever. It's like, "Well, I can come and do that, but that's not really my goal for what I'm working towards for the patients." Sometimes they see us as someone to assist them in their job.

It is important to note that not all five occupational groups engaged in doing another's "nonmedical" tasks. For instance, physicians never helped others by performing nonmedical or unskilled tasks, largely because of their status in the hospital hierarchy, their ability to remain away from the bedside, and their role as the managers or directors of the health-care team.[11] Ironically, despite their low status in the hospital, social workers rarely helped other groups carry out such tasks, as their "nonmedical" knowledge allowed them to avoid some of the "dirty" work done at the bedside. In a similar twist of the status hierarchy, occupational, physical, and speech therapists performed such tasks for others more often than social workers. While OPS therapists may have had more status and power than social workers, the fact that on the floor they sometimes performed this type of boundary work reveals a status hierarchy held together by looser ties than one may initially think.

Nonmedical tasks were most frequently performed by respiratory therapists and nurses, both of whom were most visibly and continuously present at the bedside. For nurses, this has compelling structural and symbolic implications. Nurses are still positioned as the "eyes and hands" of physicians, and regardless of their educational credentials and widening technical skills and responsibilities on the floor (which for some is evidence of work intensification without any real gains for nurses), they remain most vulnerable to the demands of other occupational groups, not just physicians.[12] Furthermore, nurses thought of themselves (and were perceived by others) as fulfilling a mediating and hands-on role that left them vulnerable to requests from practitioners who might be feeling pressured by adverse working conditions or other external circumstances.[13] Respiratory therapists and nurses could rarely avoid or ignore requests from other groups, and the frequency with which they were involved in this type of boundary work highlights their ambiguous status in the occupational hierarchy.

Transgressing the Diagnostic Line

Medical practice is uncertain and relies on practitioners' clinical experience, intuition, hunches, and insight, despite all the scientific advancements that guide it.[14] "I believe that about 15 percent of what I do is evidence-based medicine," an attending oncologist explained, "and beyond evidence-based medicine, I like to use the term 'insight-based medicine.' So I would estimate that about 85 percent of what I do is insight-based medicine, which is always a little bit hazardous statistically." Across the groups, most of the practitioners I spoke with agreed that in ideal circumstances, an evidence-based practice guided their work, but much of what they did was based on the "art" of health care, and this is where knowledge, diagnosis, and treatment can become a contested terrain, as I learned in the ICU.[15]

ICUs feel like big fish tanks. Everything is glass, and it is all visible from any one point within the unit unless someone closes the curtains of a patient's room. In each small room, a single patient lies on a bed surrounded by a variety of machinery and monitors. One afternoon, I accompanied Rich, a respiratory therapist, as he conducted his round of treatments and ventilator check-ups. We arrived at a patient who was sedated and intubated; he looked as if he was in a deep sleep.

Shortly, what began as a routine conversation between a physician and Rich quickly turned into a debate over whether a certain ventilator setting was appropriate for this patient. The physician wanted to remove the patient from the ventilator the next day and insisted that, given certain lab values, the ventilator setting he had prescribed was best until then.

After listening patiently, Rich firmly told the physician that he had treated this patient for a while and that, based on his progress, Rich's adjustments would get him off the ventilator more quickly and safely. The physician would not budge, and their technical conversation became more heated. Rich started citing studies in support of his position and proudly said that even the pulmonary physicians in the other ICUs came to him because of his knowledge and experience. "I can pick up on stuff just by looking at him breathe that a lot of people can't," Rich said confidently.

Nonetheless, the physician said that "the team" (in this case, the residents and attending) had decided to follow their protocol and that Rich ought to carry out the order. "OK, doc, I'll do [it], but you know I am right about this one."

The atmosphere was tense as everyone parted ways. Rich seemed bothered, but he did not "lose it." As he told me later that day, "You gotta pick your battles. I tried, but this one didn't work the way it should have."

The physician ultimately prevailed not because he knew more but because he pulled rank. While this instance was negotiated informally, similar situations have led to formal actions such as an incident report, which most practitioners wish to avoid, given the bureaucratic and professional implications for all involved. Through boundary work, more serious conflict between Rich and the physician was averted with "no hard feelings." Above all, Rich's transgression of the diagnostic boundary was less confrontational because while he challenged the physician's protocol, he decided that it would not harm the patient. This was not a battle that Rich deemed worth fighting beyond the tense verbal exchange—an exchange that shows how diagnostic knowledge is open to challenges, even from those on the technical side of the boundary divide.[16]

Practitioners who dealt with social, psychological, and family issues frequently engaged in this type of boundary work. A social worker recalled a physician who routinely (and incorrectly) diagnosed child neglect:

> There was a particular doctor who wanted to call Child Protective Services at the drop of a hat for neglect. One time I got in a small debate with her because there was a family that lived up near the

[state] border and they had been bad in the past about coming for
clinic visits. The patient had cystic fibrosis. . . . I had talked to them
and talked them into coming here to be seen. So, they had been
coming, they made it to a couple visits like they were supposed
to but she [the physician] was still in that mind frame [where]
they hadn't been doing the right thing. So she was saying that if
they didn't show up for their appointment that I was to call CPS
and report child neglect, and I said, "Well, what if it's because it's
snowing up there? They live way up in the mountains on this little
hill. If it's snowing and the roads aren't safe, you don't want them
to come." She said, "Yes, I do, you call CPS anyway." I said, "You
call them." She was very dictatorial; I used to call her the Gestapo.
She wanted me to go evaluate another family because the mother
had tattoos, which she thought could be a problem and a sign of
neglect! I said to her, "Well, there's no evidence that the child is not
being taken care of." So I just started joking with her: "Oh, it's the
tattoos factor . . ."

I found that social workers often reaffirmed occupational boundaries while
asserting some degree of authority regardless of their marginal and subordinate positions by maintaining that medical practitioners did not have
the knowledge to make psychosocial diagnoses.[17] Social workers satirized
and underscored the flaws in the logic employed by physicians (and, less
often, by others, like nurses) for calling child protective services (as unrea-
sonable) or miscounseling patients (as uneducated). It was hard for social
workers to ignore the devaluation of their knowledge and expertise, and
they frequently recalled such "atrocity stories" or insisted that other practitioners refrain from dictating how they addressed the psychosocial needs
of patients and families.[18] As the social worker above confided to me, she
had "put this physician in [her] place" and "she hardly got pushy like that
again."

   No group was exempt from engaging in this type of boundary work. For
instance, respiratory therapists were no strangers to cases in which they
viewed another practitioner's actions as intrusions into their own jurisdiction. As Leah explained:

There are problems a lot of times, like in the ICU, where they
[nurses] may make changes on the ventilator, where we feel they

shouldn't be touching the machine because they haven't been trained in how to operate it, and we find that they do make mistakes and it's better to leave that for us to do. . . . And the same with doctors, we have problems with them. They make a change and they don't necessarily know about ventilators, so . . . that is tiring, but that is the way it is.

A pediatric nurse shared the following account of how physicians did not always have the last word or prevail in determining a course of treatment:

He [the patient] had the surgery and his pain was out of control—it was off-the-charts out of control! So I went to the charge nurse, who suggested that I go to our clinical nurse specialist who is a pain specialist. I then called the doctor: "Can we get a consult from the pain clinic?" The answer from him was no. Then I said, "I need pain med orders for him [the patient]," and he said, "No, he should be fine." Then he [the physician] wasn't coming up when he promised, so I called him again, and I called his resident. His resident didn't care. When the attending came to the floor, our nurse specialist was there to back me up. He said, "We are not calling the pain service. . . ." Well, when the pain service came by before the ortho docs got there, we kind of curbsided him. We said, "Hey, what do you think about this med in this dose? We think it would be safe, based on this research, and we have used it before, so that we can start controlling his [the patient's] pain." So when we went to the ortho doc, we [the nurses] knew—we hadn't officially consulted, but we knew—what the safe medication dose was for this patient and we could back that up. So we could go to them [the doctors] educated and [able to say] this is what he [the patient] can handle weight-wise, age-wise, etc. The physician was going, "Well, this isn't what we do, blah, blah, blah," and [I] told the attending, "Well, here's the problem and this is what we need to do," and that is how it got solved.

This nurse and her colleagues went to great lengths to rectify what she believed was the physician's incorrect diagnosis of her patient's pain level. They avoided escalating the initial conflict because the nurse's assertive transgression did not fundamentally threaten the status of the physician, even though his opinion did not prevail and he eventually signed off on the nurse's (educated) medical advice.

Once again, not all groups engaged in diagnostic transgressions to the same extent, nor did they all equally prevail when doing so. Respiratory therapists and OPS therapists reported more boundary transgressions than social workers, physicians, and nurses. And though physicians reported fewer challenges to their knowledge and authority, they did not always get their way vis-à-vis other occupations. When other groups could make the case for how physicians were "out of their league" or could offer evidence to support their "untrained" trespassing, the diagnostic boundary was neither absolute nor unyielding. Given the interdependent work required by patient care, other occupational groups are exposed to (and in many cases hold) the very skills, knowledge, and experience that physicians claim to own exclusively, and thus boundary work can alter the course of health-care provision more often than we might imagine from macroanalyses of professionalism.[19]

Dismissing Others' Recommendations

A third type of boundary work that practitioners engaged in was dismissing the recommendations of others. In Hospital General, many things actually went "unnoticed" as practitioners sometimes turned a blind eye to others' work practices, even when they disagreed with them or knew that care protocols had not been explicitly followed.[20]

One morning, Dr. Lewis and I entered the pediatric unit, where she grabbed a chart and checked some lab results on a computer before heading to a patient's room. After an assertive knock on the door, she opened it to find a young child and his mother on the bed, watching cartoons. "Bryan, do you mind if we lower the volume? I need to listen to your lungs and heart."

Dr. Lewis talked to him while monitoring his vitals and his oxygen levels. As she was getting ready to leave the room, Dr. Lewis said, "OK, Bryan, you keep having those nutritional shakes that I ordered for you."

The mother said, "Actually, Dr. Lewis, he is not having the ones you said. The nurse brought a different brand. . . . I think it's the generic brand."

"Oh, he should be having the kind I ordered because I like the brand stuff. I'll take care of it."

Bryan's nurse, Kerry, was unavailable; deciding not to wait for her, Dr. Lewis wrote another order for the "right stuff" before we left to see another patient.

On a subsequent day, I was in the pediatric unit again, following Kerry. She was Bryan's nurse again, since the unit tries to keep patients with the same nurse as much as possible to ensure continuity of care (known as primary nursing).[21] When Kerry and I went to see him, she took his vitals and gave him medication while he sat transfixed by the television. Before leaving, Kerry said, "Bryan, don't forget to take that," pointing to the nutritional supplement on his bedside table.

Outside the room, I asked Kerry if she provided the generic or "the brand stuff." "Oh," she replied, immediately recognizing what I was referring to. "You were here the other day with Dr. Lewis. Well, that's the generic stuff. Dr. Lewis always wants the other stuff but you know they are all the same and the pharmacy sends that one, so . . ."

As we sat by the nurses' station while she charted, I asked, "So, you don't have a problem with her asking you every time to order the brand stuff?"

"It's a long story," Kerry sighed, "but I've tried in the past and now I just ignore it because it's not worth it. . . . Like I said, I call in her order, this is what they send, this is what I give the patient. . . . The pharmacy won't send the brand one. I've done my job. . . . She can be a stickler about some of these things." As the day continued, Kerry made sure that Bryan took his nutritional supplement, though it was not the "brand" one his doctor ordered.

"Dismissing," a common type of boundary work, helped to smooth out daily disagreements and differences among practitioners. Kerry and Dr. Lewis both behaved as one would have expected them to, acting systematically on protocol (i.e., physician writes order, nurse carries it out), but neither of them made a big fuss over the patient getting the generic supplement. This dismissal was predicated on a common understanding that ignoring another's request was inconsequential; the patient was not at risk and would get what he needed. Boundary work of this sort required knowledge and experience that practitioners relied on to judge the potential consequences of their actions; in dismissing, one must not risk professional status and reputation by affecting perceptions of one's competency and overall work performance. Finally, dismissing occurred when practitioners had performed a task but circumstances beyond their control had produced a different outcome (e.g., in the case of the nurse, "I have put in the order as the physician wrote it and the pharmacy sent the generic instead"). All in all, when it is reasonable, this type of boundary work effectively staves off conflict and makes things work on the floor. While dismissing others' recommendations embodies a way of managing strained interactions, it also involves pushing back: it dignifies one's decision making in response to another's authority, and is a dialectical process of accepting and rejecting the status hierarchy.

Another way this boundary work becomes evident is when a practitioner dismisses an intrusion into their area of expertise by deciding that a particular request (such as a demand for action) is inappropriate. A respiratory therapist, Craig, explained:

> I'm discussing with the nurse that this patient doesn't need a treatment because they are not wheezing at all and they're short of breath, but it's a heart condition, not a lung condition, and they want me to give this medication and I'm saying this patient doesn't need it, it's not going to fix anything. . . . Some doctors or nurses think that it does, so they want it and they push it. Usually, the RT, if they figure out it's not even worth it unless it's harmful, you won't do it. Or, "OK, I'll just give it." So it's like you are just doing it for them and you don't want to be condescending having to explain all that . . . so you just let it go.

While the other two types of boundary work were likely to involve some degree of conflict, dismissing others most often avoided it altogether. Further, the RT's dismissing helped him reaffirm his sense of expertise by highlighting the nurse's lack of knowledge in the area. Through boundary work, groups that regularly interact with each other reinforce the professional self while buffering it from the political, social, and emotional costs of conflict on the floor.

I was reminded of this once again in labor and delivery one day. Tamara, a junior nurse, was caring for a patient who had delivered her baby during the night shift. At mid-morning, Tamara asked Susan, the social worker, if she could check in on her patient. Susan was a veteran social worker with a caustic tongue and a somewhat intimidating demeanor. Her face showed the emotional toll that her job had taken over the years, and she "could not wait to retire." As we stood at the nurses' station, I sensed a confrontation brewing as Tamara and Susan talked.

As Tamara asked for a patient evaluation, Susan repeatedly asked her why, given there had been no request for a formal referral. As it turned out, the patient was "in her mid-twenties and this is child number five." Tamara said emphatically, "You have to talk to her and make her see that this is not right."

Susan looked at the nurse incredulously. "Well, let me see," she said. "Do the children show any signs of abuse or neglect? Or maybe you think she is psychologically unstable or something—"

"No, no," Tamara interrupted. "Some of her kids are from different fathers, and if she keeps having them like this . . . and obviously she doesn't know how to take care of herself, if you know what I mean."

At this point, Susan's expression turned blank, and she began filling out forms from her folder. After Tamara repeated her concerns, Susan responded in a monotone, saying that she (Susan) could enter a formal referral. Then she simply walked away.

Undeterred, Tamara went to the patient herself, with the main purpose of "educating her a little bit." The patient was unmoved—as was Susan, who still had not seen the woman when the shift ended hours later.

While the exchange could have easily escalated into more than a professional dispute, the social worker's indifference to the nurse's request left occupational and moral boundaries intact. Susan made it clear that Tamara had no authority over her work or the patient's lifestyle; the nurse had "crossed the line" in some moral or ethical sense—something that social workers prided themselves in avoiding and considered an important aspect of their professionalism.

Practitioners across groups dismissed others' recommendations or practices on a regular basis; yet, there are patterns characterizing each group's frequency to dismiss that rested on the social organization of work in the hospital. Ultimately, being able to dismiss others required a believable level of competency in a specific domain of problems and in techniques to solve them effectively.[22] Physicians were the practitioners who most frequently dismissed others' recommendations; yet, this was less obvious when they interacted with social workers with whom they did not share domains of expertise and skills. Similarly, OPS therapists could dismiss others with impunity, given their education and skills in an identifiable area of rehab work compared with the remaining groups. Ironically, social workers could often dismiss others in an environment where biomedical science was the dominant currency if those practitioners ventured into the domains of psychosocial and emotional work, which they frequently did. Finally, nurses and RTs were the least likely to dismiss others. For nurses in particular, dismissing others was difficult because management (charge nurses and unit managers) was always present to ensure their prompt compliance with the recommendations and orders of other practitioners. Still, even if the knowledge domains of RNs and RTs were considered more limited and less exclusive, both groups could still work boundaries in this manner under the right circumstances.

The Work of Boundary Work

Several points are important in my discussion of the three types of boundary work. While boundary work is an individual act, it is collectively enforced and sanctioned; it ought not to be misinterpreted as a "personal" style or issue between two or more practitioners. All three types evidenced patterns that vary in relation to occupational status, and they were practiced similarly by members of practitioner groups. Further, boundary work is an occupation's way of coping and dealing with certain realities of work, especially the need to coordinate varying practitioner roles within the occupational hierarchy. Boundary work embodies not only conflict but also the cooperative repair work necessary to minimize institutionalized inequality and "get things done and make things work."

Each type of boundary work is characterized by specific issues and implications. At the core of the practice of doing someone's "nonmedical" tasks are the strained working conditions that compel practitioners to take shortcuts when faced with heavy workloads and feeling overextended; that is, conditions that can put patient care at risk. On the other hand, at the core of diagnostic boundary transgressions is a disagreement over occupational competency in a particular area of professional practice. Here, as Andrew Abbott suggests, the implications extend from claiming expert knowledge on behalf of one's status to convincing others that one can reliably apply that knowledge in treating a specific (health) problem.[23] Finally, at the core of dismissing another's recommendation is an invocation of authority that goes unheard or not acted upon.[24] Dismissing is thus not so much about unfavorable working conditions or who can competently deploy knowledge and skills, but rather about retaining control in light of status conflicts in a particular situation.

Boundary work, as a series of situational challenges, could be characterized as a form of "floor politics" that typically takes place away from the desks of top bureaucratic echelons and administrators. As a respiratory therapist told me after a long shift, "sometimes we get the perception that maybe [nurses are] trying to take over our job and vice versa." The RT added that doctors were likewise concerned about nurses covering the same ground: "Sometimes they [physicians] feel threatened in their field." Day in and day out in Hospital General, occupational roles and interoccupational relations are routinely contested, but through boundary work the status hierarchy is ultimately reinforced *as it is breached*. Boundary work reflects the dynamic nature of professional exclusion; that is, how occupational jurisdictions can be crossed, though not substantially transformed. While these transgressions may not amount to much structurally, they are meaningful for practitioners because they inform and inspire alternatives to the hierarchy of the health-care workplace. They reflect the possibility of a "new professionalism."[25] This professionalism would reflect the transformation of the current hierarchy into more egalitarian partnerships among occupational groups and with the people they serve.[26]

Yet, a serious obstacle to this transformation is how the boundary work I have discussed relates to an ideology of caring. Given workplace pressures (such as increasing numbers of patients amid short staffing), boundary work is characterized by practitioners minimizing or setting aside their status and power differences because they are united by an ideology of caring; that is, practitioners acting in what they consider the best interests of their patients, whether that means caring *about* them (performing one's job as best one can) or caring *for* them (performing the tasks that constitute emotive caring). All three types of boundary work invoke one version of caring or the other as the ideological basis of the boundary transgression. In other words, in none of the boundary work I observed did practitioners say, for example, "I am challenging your diagnosis because I wish to challenge your power, status, or privilege," or "Even though I am performing your nonmedical tasks, don't think I'm relinquishing my power, status, or privilege," or "I'm ignoring what you told me because I resent your power, status, or privilege." Rather, all the practitioners engaged in boundary work because they were sincerely concerned for their patient's well-being and this is how to get things done in a strained hospital workplace.

In this context, an ideology of caring informs consent to the status hierarchy while obscuring how it undermines and minimizes the very acts of caring used to justify it. Each type of boundary work analyzed above prioritizes biomedical science and intervention over the caring dimension of health care, and each practitioner group is evaluated or judged against this standard. Boundary work gets "the caring stuff done," but without confronting how caring continues to be marginalized when status is conferred within the hospital. Indeed, boundary work constitutes a point at which professionalism and caring subtly intersect, where the balance struck is least intended yet likely the strongest. As we shall see, when the issue of unionism came up among practitioners (either because I asked about it or as I observed them during the course of a busy shift), professionalism and caring became much more contested, revealing vexing divisions within Hospital General.

Chapter 7

Unions: "The Elephant in the Room"

It is one thing to be underpaid, and it's one thing to be overworked, but it is another thing to be underpaid, overworked, and not appreciated!
—RESPIRATORY THERAPIST

URING my fieldwork, a highly visible and contentious battle between the hospital administration and the nurses' union rocked Hospital General. After more than a year of negotiations, the nurses' union claimed an impasse and called members to vote on a twenty-four-hour strike. With heightened tension and increasing publicity from local press coverage, a majority of nurses voting approved a walkout. Upon hearing the news, hospital administrators filed an injunction, arguing that the strike was illegal, and they secured part-time staffing from for-profit agencies that specialize in recruiting nurses, respiratory therapists, and other health-care workers to provide bedside care. When a judge ruled the strike was illegal, negotiations resumed under an atmosphere of suspicion and distrust.

The feeling on the floor was somewhat tense, although people acted as if it was business as usual. Speaking with nurses, I heard about the routine issues of patient complaints, physician unavailability, short staffing, and equipment breaking down, but their most urgent concern was whether they would strike. One nurse in the recovery unit told me that the hospital's proposal might benefit younger nurses and new recruits, but it would disadvantage older and senior nurses, given that one of the issues on the table was retirement benefits. A letter signed by several thousand nurses and sent to the administration supported the union and its efforts to negotiate a new contract that would protect new hires and retain their "ability to provide safe patient care." According to this memo, the union was concerned about three main recruitment and retention issues: adequate raises, pension and benefit protections, and fair promotions and in-hospital transfer policies. The union also wanted the negotiations to address topics related to patient care, such as the enforcement of specific staffing ratios, the introduction of new technology (which the nurses feared could be used to override their professional judgment or to replace them altogether), and "paid time off" (which the RNs objected to because it forced them to come to work sick, thus putting their patients at risk).

As autumn arrived, a compromise was reached, and the union secured a new short-term contract. Yet, during the dispute, Hospital General was being evaluated by a credentialing agency, and their assessment was negative. As a top administrator of patient care explained to me, the main issues cited in the surveyors' report were the labor dispute, a hostile working environment, and noticeable discontent among nurses in specialty units. Viewing it as "the perfect storm," this administrator suggested that had the union not created "this long and unnecessary" dispute, and had a "small, disgruntled group of nurses" not gotten the surveyors' ears, the hospital would have received a better evaluation. Though the atmosphere had calmed down, and people on the floor and in the administration had "moved on," everyone knew it was a temporary truce until the next round of negotiations for a new contract.

While health-care practitioners have long courted professional associations as their collective representatives, the appeal of unionism has grown steadily over the past half century. In California, nurses have been at the forefront of labor activism against increasing nurse-patient ratios and cutbacks on benefits, retirement, and pensions.[1] Nationally, they have organized against potential legislation that would impede nurses in nonformal, semimanagerial positions (such as charge nurses) from becoming union members.[2] Since the 1990s, physician residents in some medical centers on the East Coast have successfully concluded their unprecedented drives to unionize, prompting much controversy and disagreement among physicians nationally.[3] Others, like social workers, still debate in professional conferences and forums whether they should pursue lobbying or unionization to advance their occupational goals and professional status in the context of managed care.[4]

It is possible that with more women entering medicine, attitudes toward unionization, professionalism, and the caring ideal may change. For instance, some data suggest a gender gap, with women holding more favorable views toward unionization and socialized health-care services.[5] Likewise, some of the largest nurses' unions, such as the California Nurses Association, the Massachusetts Nurses Association, and the New York State Nurses Association, have been quite outspoken in their support for more regulation of HMOs, a change toward a more equitable and just distribution of health services, and the protection of provider working conditions, which they see as ethically linked to patients' rights.[6] For physicians, nurses, respiratory therapists, social workers, and OPS therapists who have grappled with professionalism and caring, unionization is the "pink elephant in the room."

Unionization has historically been controversial among nurses and other health-care practitioners since not only bread-and-butter economic issues are at stake but also ethical ones. Debates over unionization highlight the tensions between professionalism and caring in an organizational context that challenges those very ideals. Understandably, the practitioners I interviewed held strong opinions about whether they supported or opposed unionization and actions such as striking. At Hospital General, I found that practitioners on opposite sides of the union divide relied on similar arguments to justify their positions. Here, the intersection of the professional self and caring was most salient but also, unsurprisingly, most volatile, as these ideals were resolved *only for those on one or the other side of the debate*. Recall that boundary work is an informal process of teamwork at best, and it upholds caring in ways that challenge professional jurisdictions but never replace them. Instead, it represents the floor politics that "gets things done" without transforming the organizational status hierarchy or the subordinate status of caring. Unionization, conversely, is a formal alternative to teamwork, insofar as it unites caring and professionalism. Yet it does so only at the cost of another division—that of how practitioners politicize caring and professionalism. In the case of boundary work, the ideological nature of professionalism and caring is subdued, submerged within the apolitical discourse of floor conflicts. With unionism, the ideological nature of both could not be more vivid, more public, and more incriminating. With unionism, professionalism and caring are estranged along "partisan" lines; it is an ongoing impasse that haunts health care in Hospital General, and arguably in the United States as well.

It is worth noting that only physicians (attending and resident) were not unionized at Hospital General, as nurses, respiratory therapists, social workers, and OPS therapists were represented by different unions to which practitioners paid dues. Whereas OPS therapists were clearly ambivalent in weighing the "pros and cons" of unionism, social workers and RTs expressed few reservations and unequivocally supported unionization. But it was among physicians and nurses where there was a clear split between those opposing and supporting unionization. And it may be among these practitioners that the professional-caring conflict is most significant, as these are the largest occupational groups in Hospital General and the most influential in defining, establishing, and reinforcing the parameters of health-care debate and provision.

Sitting on the Fence: OPS Therapists

Most OPS therapists were either unsure of what to make of unionization or claimed to know little about it. "I think we have a small union," said one occupational therapist. "It's called UTPE or something, but it's not a formal union. . . . I really don't have a strong opinion on that. I know some people do. . . . I'm kind of indifferent." She added, "I guess people are working towards getting us more involved, but I'm not going to the meetings and getting involved in that. . . . I'm not going to be like, "No, thanks," to the union, but I'm happy and I really don't feel that strongly about changing anything. . . . I don't have strong feelings about it. . . . To be honest, I don't know much about the union stuff."

Larry, a speech therapist, knew little about the union, saying that it might be unnecessary for practitioners like him:

> It's the first time I've ever had to belong to a union. For the first year and a half, I knew I was paying union dues, but I really didn't know anything else, [such as] that I even had to fill out paperwork to where I would give information for my union. . . . None of us kind of knew this, so I guess it wasn't just me. . . . I don't see what the benefits from the union are. . . . The first two years and a half, I didn't get anything, and then we got like a 2 percent raise. . . . I don't know. . . . I've never been in a situation where I needed it. . . . I don't feel that in this day and age, at least for my job level and people like me, a union is that necessary, but I guess it doesn't

really bother me that I belong to the union so . . . I kinda go back and forth on the issue.

All things considered, OPS therapists recognized that unionization tested their professional values and calling to care, but they were also aware of the potential gains they could enjoy through union representation. "I have mixed feelings about it, actually," a physical therapist explained:

> On the one hand, I think that maybe unions are not appropriate for physical therapists, getting back to the idea of professionalism. I don't know that a job like that is appropriate for a union to be representing. On the other hand, we are working and we are working for someone and that someone may or may not always have our best interest in mind, so maybe it's good to have a selective group who does have our best interests in mind. But then on the flip side of that is 'What's the union really done for PTs, besides take their dues?" So I have pretty mixed feelings about the whole thing. . . . I can kind of see both sides, and I can see a group of workers not wanting to be taken advantage of, but at the same time, at whose expense? At the patients' expense? So, again, I have very mixed feelings about that.

The PT said that he himself would not walk out, given his commitments to his patients, but immediately followed that with, "Then again, I could, if I really saw a compelling reason," such as being made to see more patients than humanly possible.

This ambivalence over what unionism implied about their professionalism and caring ideals also characterized the practitioners' views toward striking. While a strike might compromise the health and recovery of their patients if not carefully planned and executed, they also believed that gaining leverage over the hospital administration could benefit them and possibly their patients. As Tina, a physical therapist, put it:

> It really depends on the issue and the situation. It's not like, "Yeah, you should always strike," or "No, you should never strike." I think if things are so bad that you're compromising all these things that in the end can hurt your patients, then that [striking] might in the long run be a better thing, even if you are putting some people at

risk in the short term. . . . You have to look at the big picture, and it might be such a bad situation that it's putting people [patients and practitioners] at risk for working in bad conditions. At the same time, if it's for two thousand dollars or something like that, or for a 1 percent pay raise, going on strike doesn't make any sense and the risks to patients are too many for just that. I really don't want to say one way or the other. I think it depends on the severity of the issue. It would depend on the situation.

The ambivalence of OPS therapists is interesting, given that their work rarely involves critical care or life-and-death situations, and their potential absence from the bedside was unlikely to result in serious threats to patient well-being. Perhaps this uncertainty reflects the divided character of their professional self; they are independent contractors of a sort, who are at the same time hired employees working under the shadow of physicians. Social workers and respiratory therapists seldom felt such contradictions from their experiences in Hospital General.

Solidarity Forever? Social Workers and Respiratory Therapists

Practically all the social workers supported unionization and striking, given what little power they had with the hospital administration in shaping their working conditions. And though they were dissatisfied with the current union's ability to negotiate successfully, it was better than nothing. Helen was adamant about the need for representation: "I've seen what [managers have] done to people in the lab that didn't have a union, like not scheduling them for more than two weeks out so they couldn't make any plans. . . . A union gives you some protection and legal recourse, and considering how this hospital administration works, I feel that [the union is] very important for our protection."

The promise of protection was even more significant to social workers because they felt that they held considerably less status and power than other practitioners with comparable (or lower) levels of education such as OPS therapists or nurses. As one social worker I interviewed explained:

I am a member and I believe in being represented so that we can get the benefits that we deserve. . . . We're thought of as the bottom of the barrel. . . . We're in there "raking out the muck" of situations and we should be compensated. . . . We have master's degrees. We're professionals. How many RNs just have a two-year degree? We have a four-year degree, plus [a] minimum [of] two years more, plus we're licensed and that's another four-year process. We're licensed in this state to do psychotherapy; I can hang out my own shingle and do private practice. . . . There's some power in having the union representation, especially because we're viewed as the little guy here. . . . In a big medical institution like this one, it's a benefit.

Social workers often expressed discontent with their low pay and meager perks, especially as well-educated professionals who are the first to respond to the caring needs of patients and practitioners alike (and compared to nurses, whom they consider less trained and less specialized). Their feeling marginalized and disempowered in Hospital General led social workers to be even more critical of the administration's intentions and policies than the RTs were.

Even though some social workers held reservations about how striking might impact the well-being of patients, a majority saw no problems with walking the walk. "I would definitely go on strike," one social worker defiantly said. He then detailed why:

Three years ago, nurses had their contract renewed, and they got about 24 percent a year [in increased pay] over a three-year period. Then it came to the next year, when our union was fighting for us, and we got 3 percent, 2 percent, 3 percent, and they [the administration] said, "I'm sorry, that's all you can have, that's all we have." We were saying, 'But gosh, look at the nurses, they got so much." That's the kind of fighting words where we need to say it is about the salary and it is about the insult, about the value you're placing on social workers in this setting versus the value you're placing on nurses in this setting. . . . Under those circumstances, I would say, "Yes, let's go out on strike." . . . Everyone knows that if nurses went on strike, you cripple a hospital, but if social workers go on strike, it's not like, "Oh my god, we're going to have to shut down the hospital." Nobody's going to die. . . . Nurses can bring the rotation of the hospital to a halt, and it would be great for us if we could have the same effect.

Because their jobs did not involve direct medical treatment, social workers felt that striking would not threaten patients or even the overall functioning of the hospital. Ironically, most of them conceded that their absence would "hardly be noticed." Perhaps recognizing this, they realized that striking was not the best approach to stalled negotiations, though they considered it a "necessary evil" if push came to shove.

Respiratory therapists who favored unionization argued that without it hospital management would "walk all over" them.[7] Although they did not think union representation contradicted their professionalism or caring ideals, their support of it signaled their devalued status as "mere" technical workers who nonetheless would like more colleague recognition. "I have always felt that unions were a good thing," one RT explained:

> I think that unions balance things out: they balance out the tendency of owners and managers to exploit other employees. . . . It's a good thing [because] the union has the ability to get people together and put their interests on the table as one. . . . In the last three or four years, things have improved greatly for us [RTs] because of the union. The union sent some people in who actually seem to understand what we do and are able to take our thoughts and ideas and get the administration to consider our needs.

Viewing the union as protection from the hospital administration, another RT concurred:

> Every advancement we have ever gotten here, we had to go to the union for it. . . . It is one thing to be underpaid, and it is one thing to be overworked, but it is another thing to be underpaid, overworked, and not appreciated! That's what we've been. . . . The union to me has been fantastic. . . . I would strike because it is about what is fair. That's what it comes down to. I don't know why that is a hard concept for anyone to grasp. The CEO of this hospital took a $250,000 bonus last year while he cut many jobs across units and departments in Hospital General. . . . It's unfortunate we have to have the union to fight for us, it's really unfortunate we have to fight for it, but that is the reality.

Most RTs saw unionization as the best way to improve working conditions and compensation without compromising their professional and caring ideals. They were more uncertain, however, when it came to the issue of striking. Just over half of those I interviewed stated that they would strike "within reason"; that is, only if patient issues and contingencies were thoroughly addressed and if the reasons for striking benefited RTs and patients alike. As one RT explained:

> I would strike if, for example, they [management] had decided to have one therapist on per shift running around putting out fires throughout the hospital. That's not only bad for the RT who is having to run around but it's also a major safety issue that affects patients directly. . . . That's putting patients' lives at risk and that's not right. Something like that goes against our do no harm commitment and it's plain wrong. To me, that's an ethics issue and that's a moral issue. I would strike on that because it's morally and ethically an issue affecting us and our patients.

In this case of professionalism and caring aligning, just under half of RTs plainly opposed striking, feeling that it would harm their patients. For those who rejected the idea of striking, the following was typical:

> You can't do it [striking]! That's not our mission. . . . That's unthinkable to me, though it is probably legal. It defies the mission of what health-care providers do. I hope I don't ever have to see that. . . . If I were the consumer or patient, I would have no respect for it. . . . If you've been a patient, you can understand how essential health-care providers are. . . . I just can't even imagine it. I've never been on a ventilator with my life at risk, [but] I've had surgery and I know it hurts an awful lot and I was just so thankful for my staff.

Another RT agreed, saying that she couldn't see herself going on strike: "It's been proven that nurses can't manage ventilators and neither can doctors. . . . They [nurses and doctors] don't know how to set ventilators, they don't know how take care of them, and it could cause loss of life and nothing is worth that!"

Respiratory therapists who rejected striking were likely to see it as further undermining their already fragile professional self while contradicting the caring impulses they held.

Split Down the Middle: Physicians and Nurses

I was not surprised when physicians I spoke with objected to unionization. "I think it is a bad idea!" one physician exclaimed. "It interferes with the societal contract—with the patient-physician relationship." She believed that it was not appropriate for physicians to consider striking: "Are you going to tell your patients, 'Sorry, I won't be taking care of you?' I don't see how that could be reconciled. . . . *Taking care of patients is not like other jobs*. . . . They [patients] don't want to be *treated like a job to be done*" (emphasis added).

Just as caring can be seen as resisting the objectification of patients, many physicians opposed unionization for the same reason: it treated patients like a commodity produced on an assembly line. Many felt that unionization and striking contradicted the ethos and practice of caring. Dr. Saunders said:

> As a physician, you vow to help the lives of your patients. It is what they call a fiduciary relationship . . . you are looking out for that other person. I don't think it is right for doctors to go on strike and not care for patients in the hospital because that is just not right. Ethically I have a problem with that—walking out on patients when they need you to care for them because you want more money or more vacation time. I have a hard time understanding physicians who do what they do only because they have a good lifestyle or they get paid more. . . . Morally, it's a problem . . . because you don't go into medicine wanting those things. You shouldn't go into medicine wanting those things!

It was surprising, however, to find so many other physicians who did support unionization, and possibly even striking. These physicians felt that they had little say in the administrative decisions of Hospital General and that controlling their work was "a thing of the past." "I think that we should be part of a union," one physician told me as we sipped coffee before rounds. "As a resident, I felt overworked and exploited, and now that I am an attending faculty, I wish I could just tell them [residents] that it doesn't get any better. . . . They are not just being trained to be doctors, they are being trained to work under extremely adverse conditions."

While working conditions and compensation were important for physicians who supported unionization, so too was their ability to make decisions about patient care independently from hospital administration and insurance companies. Seeing their independence eroding, these physicians felt that their professional self *and* the well-being of their patients were at stake. One physician offered this dour assessment:

> If you work for a medical center like this one, you get a paycheck; your work is determined by those you work for. You see the number of patients you are told to see, your billings go through a billing group, the administration determines your pay, etc. . . . I think in the next decade, if things continue the way they are, you are going to see an increased interest in physician unions. . . . The problem is not asking for another dollar an hour. . . . You have to look at the risks. . . . If I work for St. Mary's or Hospital General and I am told at a meeting that it was decided I had to see forty patients today, not thirty, . . . that gets in the way of my professionalism. If, in another meeting, they say, "Today we decided we no longer give aspirin, so you will be fired if you prescribe aspirin to your patient," I think that is an abuse of my professionalism, too! I think there needs to be a counterweight to that and right now there isn't one. If as a single physician you go in and complain, you are told, "Thank you very much, you can find a job elsewhere." But we would have more leverage if we were part of a union.

The physicians who sensed that they would have to continue coping with deteriorating working conditions and dwindling autonomy considered unionization a viable alternative for representation vis-à-vis what seemed the unmatched power of the nonmedical administration, health-care management organizations, and government-directed health programs. For them—as it was for those who opposed unions—the "bottom line" was their ability to reclaim a calling to care and to redeem their professional self. As one physician explained, striking gives workers a lot of leverage, but it is not a compelling option for physicians since "they are a little bit held hostage to their jobs." Despite this conundrum, physicians who supported unionization contemplated how striking might not necessarily endanger their ideals. Dr. McCormick said, "I think we should have the right to strike within reason, sure!" He elaborated on what "within reason" might mean:

> We are not going to walk away from a critically ill patient, but I
> don't see any reason why my clinic can't be closed for a couple of
> days, and those patients reappointed in three or six months. Or why
> noncritical patients can't be sent to another institution or wait if no
> threat is posed to their health. Yes, they [patients] are going to be
> angry. Yes, they are going to feel like their own rights are violated,
> but I think it is a matter of fairness and justice. I know other places
> that strike still manage to keep the basic necessities running.

Dr. McCormick pointed out that when power-plant workers strike, "they
don't turn the power plant off. If hospital practitioners strike, we won't turn
the hospital off either! Only the nonessential services would be cut down. I
think that is very doable."

The physicians' support for unionization and striking reflected their
deepening concern that despite being highly educated and skilled, they
were becoming "just like any other worker" in the hospital. If this support
contradicted much of their image as professionals, they would counter that
unionization was also emerging as the only viable recourse they had to
stem or reverse their eroding status.

Like the physicians who opposed unionization, just under half of the
nurses felt that it compromised the professional self and caring for patients.
"Unionization is not a good thing," Kathy explained. "To the extent that
unionization fractures off into its own agenda or power trip, it may detract
from professionalism." She spelled out why she was opposed to striking:

> Striking is not a good thing for nursing because what you are doing
> is withholding not just a commodity. When a nurse strikes, they are
> withholding essential care from another person—they are with-
> holding caring. And they don't harm the institution until they have
> already harmed individuals physically and in other ways. And that is
> why I think a strike among nurses, a strike among police officers, a
> strike among fire people, is immoral, because they harm individuals
> in order to achieve their own financial means.

Conversely, nurses who supported unionization considered it the most
effective way to abate management abuse of the professional self and patient care. A veteran nurse asserted that having a union was great, because

"it's a protection from management." She had learned from experience not to trust the management:

> They claim to have our best interests at heart, but they would pay us absolutely as little as possible if they could, and they would have us working in completely unacceptable conditions if they could. The union forces them to abide by certain basic standards. . . . Because of the union, there's been a lot of pay, a lot of work hour and patient ratio improvements. . . . When I was young, I was very idealistic. I would say, "I will not abandon my patients, I will work no matter what, and I will cross the picket line!" Over the years, I've found that actually it's in the best interest of patients that we fight for good compensation and for rights for nurses! Nursing is very difficult work, the pay is not anywhere near comparable to a lot of other professions . . . The union is one of the most powerful ways to do it.

Like their physician counterparts, nurses who supported unionization believed that improving their working conditions meant better-quality care for their patients. However, they too, like physicians, hedged their support for striking. They did not think striking was inherently bad, but they supported it only if it was well planned and did not jeopardize their patients. "As long as patients are not harmed," Janet said, "I would strike, yeah!" She anticipated how the administration would respond:

> For one thing, the hospital will spend millions of dollars to bring in nurses from temp agencies; they're not actually going to let any patient suffer. They're going to reroute patients to other hospitals, they're going to discharge patients, they're not going to schedule elective surgery, etc. . . . In the long term, the positive effects that you can get from striking far outweigh any short-term negative effects. But still, it doesn't mean you do it blindly or without having second thoughts. . . . It's a really hard decision to make.

Recalling the last round of negotiations between their union and hospital administration, another nurse admitted that striking is a hard choice to face. "Taking your oath as a nurse, patient care comes first," Rose explained, "but nobody was going to harm none of the patients because what they [management] were doing was turning people away from the hospital anyway and they just rescheduled all of the patients that were getting surgery. . . . So it was very, very difficult and you don't cross the picket line if you [don't] have to, but you are always worried about it." Reflecting on the dilemma posed by unionization, Stephanie, a young nurse, recalled her agonizing decision to strike:

> We did vote to strike last year. We never did strike, thank God, and we were all praying that we wouldn't have to strike. It wasn't because we were afraid we were going to lose money. It was the fact that we were afraid for our patients not having the right care. . . . I know that they were bringing in staffing from all over to take care of patients. But you still feel responsible for your patients. So it was really scary. I think that each and every one of us was pretty concerned when it came to that, because nobody really wanted to, but we have to do these hard things in order to bring about change, and it isn't always pleasant.

Just as physicians felt that being committed to patients was central to their professionalism, nurses too expressed the same concern over what most practitioners viewed as the most radical and taboo of labor actions—striking.

For nurses and physicians who supported it, unionization embodied a defense of their workplace interests—interests that they viewed as essentially linked to the well-being of their patients. Unionization, as they conceived it, did not contradict their professional self or caring ideals; rather, they saw it as protecting and enhancing both. In contrast, those who opposed unionization argued that it was antithetical to professionalism and caring, leaving patients to suffer the consequences of untreated or maltreated medical conditions. In both cases, the rhetoric of professionalism and caring was clearly ideological, with the practitioners employing it to cast their narrow self- or occupational interests (e.g., for more control or more money) in the ennobling light of a larger public good (i.e., serving patients). And herein lies the problem: in reference to unionism, are professionalism and caring merely compatible ideologies that mask more pecuniary or status-based interests? Or, to the degree that ideologies advance enlightened self-interest (or what Alexis de Tocqueville called "self-interest properly understood"), are professionalism and caring irreconcilable except when aligned on one side or the other of the union divide?[8] Will health care in the United States be vitiated by dissension from within as those who provide it become as dismayed as the critics and public looking in?

Lastly, the views of practitioners toward unionism might be considered alongside their views toward administration politics. As I discussed in Chapter 5, the practitioners I interviewed believed that the administration held too much power, that it cared about profits more than patient care and professional integrity, and that its politics were at the root of most of their problems. Though this view was widely shared by practitioners from all occupational groups, it is most harmonious with the convictions of those who also supported unionism, as it reaffirms their belief in collective bargaining as the most effective approach for salvaging both patient care and professional integrity in the hospital. But for those who opposed unionism, one can only speculate about whether they view unions (and striking) as a worse evil or whether they believe that professional strategies (i.e., their esteemed knowledge base) and membership (i.e., occupational associations) can best counter administrative power and abuse.

While I researched this book, negotiations between the hospital and the cooks, clericals, and maintenance union led to a deadlock. One day, as I sipped coffee in the hospital's central lobby, which was bustling like any other day, these workers demonstrated outside the hospital's main entrance, their colorful signs stating the need for fair contracts. As some physicians with white coats and stethoscopes around their necks walked by, one of the demonstrators remarked, "Hey doc, you may need it [unionization] someday soon!" A couple of the young physicians looked at him in disbelief, and two others rolled their eyes and shook their heads in disapproval.

As they walked by me, one of the physicians said, "They are a nuisance." Perhaps they were. For so many practitioners in Hospital General, however, one person's nuisance was slowly but steadily becoming another's necessity.

Conclusion

A COLLEAGUE recently shared with me his experience in an emergency room of another regional hospital. It attests to the tenuous relationship between professionalism and caring I have considered in this book. Richard is seventy-five years old and had recently fallen outside his home. "I was in a hurry to make an appointment and it was at night. When I fell, I hit my head on a cement curb that stuck up about five inches from the sidewalk. My glasses flew off, and I was bleeding badly from my forehead and around my eyes." Fortunately, a young friend was there to drive Richard to his appointment; after helping him stagger into his house to survey the damage, the friend said, "We have to go to emergency *now*."

Richard had never been in an emergency room before. "My health is fine for my age, and I had not been inside a hospital as a patient for over fifty years." It was a Wednesday night, and the emergency room was not busy: perhaps five or six patients were in the waiting area. After checking in briefly and showing his HMO card, Richard was called after only ten minutes, "probably due to my age." He was bleeding rather badly and trying to stop the flow of blood as best he could when "a friendly female worker, dressed in a green top, called my name." She was the first of the six health-care workers Richard saw before checking out of emergency, and she ushered him into one of the three rooms he was to visit during his brief stay. After Richard answered a few background questions and described how the injury happened, she left, saying that her colleague would be in to see him.

Shortly, another practitioner appeared "to check me over and to see if I needed stitches and to clean me up a little. She asked if I felt OK—was I able to stand and walk, did I feel faint. She then led me to another room that was a short walk away. She was very friendly and seemed concerned about my condition." When Richard was in the new room, he was told that "Bill" would be coming to clean his wounds.

After a short wait, Bill arrived. Richard described their interaction:

> He said only about two sentences to me. The first was, "I am here to clean you up." He appeared to be in a bad mood—not friendly like the others had been. He was all business. He was not gentle around my face and [he was] actually rough using his hands. In fact, his touch caused me some discomfort. After cleaning the wounds and putting temporary bandages on them, he left, only saying, "Dr. Bibby will come to sew you up."

Before the physician arrived, the attendant who first saw Richard told him that he would need an x-ray. She walked him down to X-ray, where he was seen immediately. The x-ray technician then told Richard how to find his way back to the appropriate room. Richard waited there for "maybe twenty minutes" before Dr. Bibby arrived:

> He was very friendly, very talkative, very reassuring. He told me more about my injuries than any of the previous health-care workers I had encountered. He said, "I will have to use about seven or eight stitches on one wound and maybe three or four on another." He also told me that I had a broken nose and that he hoped it would heal without surgery. While Dr. Bibby was doing the stitching, he kept asking me, "Are you all right? Any discomfort?" When he finished, he said someone would come in to apply bandages. He also wrote a prescription for pain that I picked up before leaving the hospital.

The bandage worker arrived about fifteen minutes later. She was extremely friendly and kept telling Richard that he would be all right and that his wounds would heal in time. Before she left, Richard asked if he could go home, but she said he might have to wait for the x-ray results. "I told her I think Dr. Bibby already had them, but she told me to wait."

Richard duly waited for a while, but no one came, so he got up and wandered out. He found the friendly bandage worker, who found out that he could leave after filling out some paperwork at the check-in desk. At the desk, he was told he had to pay what his HMO plan required for use of the emergency room, and then "I was free to go."

Reflecting on his emergency room experience, Richard was somewhat amazed that he was "passed through" so many health-care professionals, given a somewhat minor emergency:

> Six health-care workers, including Dr. Bibby, took care of me. Five of them were friendly and caring, perhaps because they had the time to be. It did not seem hectic or busy that night in the emergency room. What was surprising to me was the division of labor—each worker had a highly specific task to perform. The thought struck me that I was on a factory assembly line, with each worker doing a specific job so that when I left I was able to "run" on my own and be displayed in the showroom.

As an outsider, Richard did not have any way of knowing if this assembly line was a form of teamwork. He mused on whether each of these workers had been randomly chosen to see him and whether they had been busy with other patients or sitting around waiting to be called:

> I did not get any clues about the workers being a cohesive team. Was the care I received only a product of each of these individuals doing their job, given their skills, personalities, demeanor, and the flow of traffic that night, or was it a result of conscious and cohesive teamwork organized by the hospital? Did they communicate with one another about me outside of my view? Or was my care the result of a random selection of individuals who I happened to encounter? It would have helped if I had known—if perhaps the first health- care worker I encountered had told me that I would be seen by a team tonight, that they all work together trying to provide me with the best care they can, and that consequently I would be seen by five or six members of the team before I left. My overall care was given efficiently and it was acceptable, but I do not know why. Was it because of the structure of the hospital and this emergency room, the unionization of the workers, this hospital [being] unionized, the professionalism and training of the staff, or the luck of my draw-

ing individuals who overall happened to be competent and caring professionals who had the time that night to be caring? I was never asked to evaluate the experience by the hospital administration.

For Richard, the issue was not about feeling uncared for, or not receiving expert medical attention. It was that he felt worked on in ways (like "on a factory assembly line") that made the care he received feel somewhat disassociated from those who were treating him: "If only someone had told me at the very beginning that this is what would be happening to me, I would have felt much more comfortable. Just knowing what was in store for me would have relieved the anxiety I was feeling."

Richard's experience could be considered a "best-case" scenario by most accounts, but what of the rest? What are we to make of this impasse between professionalism and caring? Can they be reconciled in ways where each is complementary to the other rather than in tension—a tension that relegates caring to a professional self as disputed and contentious as it is esteemed? These are not merely academic issues, of interest only to the student or scholar, but the daily concerns of practitioners, patients, and administrators in this and other hospitals throughout the United States. One need only walk into Hospital General and view the patient satisfaction surveys on display in every department, in every office, in every clinic to recognize the importance of professionalism and caring in the modern hospital. Similarly, these concerns are increasingly being addressed in health-care training and educational programs across the country.

It is possible to imagine various responses to this situation that are more or less compelling, but still fall short in one way or another. One obvious solution is to reintegrate caring into the ideology of professionalism, specifically under the ethos of a "calling" and the ideal of universal service.[1] That practitioners should embrace caring as part of their obligation to the larger community (of patients) is the flip side of the privileges they enjoy and the intrinsic value of their work. Yet, as the professional self we encountered in Chapter 1 reveals, this obligation has been seriously eclipsed by the status-conferring role of expertise and the hierarchical ranking of practitioners in terms of (biomedical) knowledge. As long as this situation prevails, the value of caring will continue to diminish as practitioners seek to acquire or enhance their knowledge in relation to other practitioners. As we saw in Chapter 3, caring was considered "the icing on the cake" as practitioners prioritized curative concerns or biomedical and technical interventions. Even though social workers embraced caring more than others, they were also the most marginal and possibly most understaffed group in Hospital General. OPS therapists were able to integrate caring into their rehabilitative practice, given their prestructured time with patients, yet they were the exception, as were their patients. It is highly unlikely under current conditions that physicians or nurses will enjoy such allotted time for caring as we saw in Chapter 3. Clearly "time" is of the essence when it comes to caring, but increasing staffing levels to achieve this is wishful thinking, given the cost crisis currently afflicting health care in the United States.

Another option might be to simply accept, as we saw in Chapter 3, that all practitioners care, they just do so in different ways. And while I have no reason to doubt the sincerity of those who make this claim, it redefines caring to suit one's situation and one's interests, and it fails to address that emotive caring has steadily lost ground in favor of the more high-stakes cure orientation to health care. Even if one is unconvinced by the evidence (from inpatient as well as primary care settings) that emotive caring and related behaviors improve the success of cure interventions and long-term health outcomes, a more humane system of heath care calls for more balance between these orientations.[2]

If one acknowledges the positive health outcomes that accrue from effective caring, one might reconsider caring as a skill set on its own behalf—one that requires advanced skills and knowledge that are as difficult to master as they are to deploy effectively.[3] Certainly a case could be made that even Hospital General must think caring deserves such attention, given its investment of considerable resources toward its caring workshops. But, as I argued in Chapter 4, these workshops were concerned less with helping practitioners (primarily nurses) develop caring knowledge and skills and more with reinforcing a caring ideology that held individual practitioners responsible for emotive caring and "friendly" work relations. What I mean by "caring knowledge and skills" differs somewhat from what Sioban Nelson and Suzanne Gordon argue in *The Complexities of Care*: they write that the caring skills deployed by nurses ought to be considered *as based* in biomedical science and on par with those of physicians, rather than as demonstrations of a virtue embraced by the profession but long past their usefulness.[4] While I agree with Nelson and Gordon on the science-based knowledge (whether formally acquired or held tacitly from experience) and role of these skills, I would argue that their thesis still overlooks the skills and knowledge necessary for emotive caring and that it inadvertently devalues an important dimension of caring in favor of biomedical and physical interventions. Still, even if one were to convincingly demonstrate that emotive caring skills and knowledge were of equal value as biomedical science and curative interventions, the fact is that all practitioners *and their training institutions* uphold the latter and so socialize their aspiring members to this orientation.[5]

Perhaps emotive caring ought to be the calling of another occupation that has links to the hospital but is not considered part of the "health-care team." Here I am thinking of the representatives of religious communities of faith, or perhaps resurrecting an enhanced version of the traditional "candy striper" (or perhaps a "patient buddy"), albeit someone whose training and role in the hospital as a caregiver would be acknowledged, valued, and of course, justly compensated. The balancing act of professionalism and caring could then be evaded insofar as practitioners could focus on applying strictly biomedical knowledge rather than being responsible for emotive caring. This would not, however, effectively address the conflicts that arise from the professional status hierarchy or the degree to which practitioners still have to cope with their own emotional involvement with patients and one another on a daily basis.

At another level, the hospital culture of teamwork might be a step in the direction of integrating caring with the professional self, but alas, it too falls short, as we saw in Chapter 2. Caring is nowhere to be seen in this culture, and most of the disputes over teamwork center on the status hierarchy and its discontents. And if the unofficial and informal teamwork that emerges when considering boundary work more closely resembles the ideal of care, it is an ideal of "last resort," operating through interactions that reinforce status distinctions and occupational jurisdictions while obscuring the absence of organizational support for caring.

At the core of this problem lie two features of Hospital General (and I would argue of other hospitals as well) that make it very difficult to arrive at a suitable resolution. One is that professional relations and caring are overwhelmingly framed as *individual rather than organizational challenges.*[6] Within this paradigm, it is practitioners who must change, or at least make sense of theirs and other's shortcomings, in ways that do not impugn personal motives or the integrity of their occupation. Likewise, to the degree that the professional-caring tension is recognized, and I believe that practitioners and administrators alike at least sense it, it is viewed as a problem that can be treated by heavy doses of *cultural therapy* rather than through the more difficult and threatening *structural changes* that are required. As I have shown in Chapters 2 and 4, Hospital General has engaged in intensive efforts to effect a "change of attitude" among practitioners by fostering an organizational culture that speaks to both professionalism (via teamwork) and caring (via workshops and public displays of patient surveys and the care ideal). Not only does this organizational culture fail to unite professionalism and caring in any meaningful and coherent way, but cultural tinkering minus structural changes to support it risks collegial cynicism, distrust, professional burnout, and narrow, self-serving practices. Unfortunately, most of the advice proffered to organizations these days focuses on organizational cultures and how to change or develop employee attitudes rather than how to address the structural conditions from which discontent and concerns arise. As I noted earlier, practitioners already enter health care with noble intents and a caring orientation, but these sentiments are systematically eroded by their working conditions and the lack of adequate organizational support to nourish and strengthen such sentiments.

If we move to the level of larger structural change toward a meaningful reconciliation of professionalism and caring, we will likely confront several hurdles, even as we head in a more promising direction. The option of professional unions among health-care workers has gained steam in the past few decades in the United States, but as I argued in Chapter 7, this only resolves the issue for those on one side or the other of the union debate. On the other hand, it is not surprising that the United States has flirted with socialized health care for well over half a century.[7] The reasons for this are not hard to find: they include changing working conditions and sources of employment, the constraints of managed care and rising costs of private insurance, increasing social inequality, and a growing uninsured population.[8] But even if we were to move to a single-payer, national health-care model—a utopian scenario, despite compelling agreement on its cost value and sporadic public support over the years—the examples of England and Canada raise concerns over the ongoing vulnerability of professionalism under the "new managerialism" in health care.[9] As the recent Francis Report on Britain's NHS documents in startling detail, socialized health care is no panacea to this dilemma, given government-imposed financial targets and what Max Weber once termed the "iron cage" of bureaucracy.[10]

Likewise, scholars have debated the impact of HMOs and private insurance systems in the United States and market-state systems abroad on professional autonomy, privileges, and ethics.[11] Some argue that deprofessionalization and deskilling has characterized the experience and the occupational trajectory of physicians and other occupations seeking professional standing.[12] It is undeniable that these structural and organizational pressures (mainly due to commodifying and rationalizing healthcare services) affect practitioners' discretionary powers, but it is unclear from my study how severe this is. Some scholars, like Richard Hugman, have proposed the notion of "re-professionalization" as a more accurate depiction of the post-industrial professional experience; it is a term, Hugman argues, that allows for both upgrading and degrading processes as well as for exploring how occupations attempt to acquire, maintain, or protect professional standing.[13]

Eliot Freidson argues that professionalism is a third logic for organizing work. He asserts that compared to market and bureaucratic logics, professionalism holds the most hope for ensuring the interests and well-being of occupational members and those receiving their services.[14] Others, like Celia Davies and Jane Salvage, have called for a "new professionalism" as the organizing principle in health-care services, given its potential for more egalitarian, democratic, and participatory relationships among occupational groups and between practitioners and their patients.[15] Based on recognizing a plurality of knowledges in health-care provision, this model of professionalism seeks to transcend narrow professional jurisdictions and reintegrate caring into the health-care process. Referring to Davies's seminal article on the new professionalism, Salvage writes:

> "Recognising the contribution of others to health and healing"
> means much more than doctors acknowledging that nurses or
> physiotherapists do a good job. It requires fundamental redefinition
> of the knowledge base of health care. Valuing the contribution of
> all means expanding an understanding of health care's boundaries
> far beyond the traditional confines of scientific medicine and its
> mastery, which usually constitutes medical expertise. Davies sug-

gests a fresh approach to health care knowledge that "sees it confirmed in use, that values things other than the formal and abstract,
copes with uncertainty, acknowledges the intuitive and accepts the
importance of experience . . . as something that grows and develops
from the fusion of expertise and experience and the formal and the
intuitive."[16]

Building on the weaknesses and disappointments of national health
care in countries comparable to the United States (borne out by the recent
Francis Report), the approach described by Davies and Salvage may offer
our most promising path, both in terms of an ideal system of heath care and
a blueprint for achieving it. Or, one could simply accept that professionalism and caring must always be in tension—that this is as good as it gets
and we had best live with it. But I doubt this acceptance will happen, since
scholars, practitioners, and the public would not be discussing the tension
so fervently now were they resigned to such a fate.

A Final Visit to the Hospital

On one of my last trips to Hospital General, I visited the pediatric intensive
care unit (PICU). It was a busy day in the PICU—a day in which I filled
quite a few pages in my notebook and also left with bittersweet memories
of the practitioners I met, the work they do, the patients they help, and the
challenges everyone faces in the hospital.

The PICU was arranged like any other intensive care unit, with its glass-
enclosed rooms, a main desk, and a nurses' station from where everything
was visible, including nurses, physicians, a social worker, a respiratory
therapist, and OPS therapists going about their business. What differenti-
ated the PICU from other intensive care units was not only the marine-
themed paintings and the colorful designs on the walls but also how young
and small its patients were. On all my visits to the PICU, despair followed
me as I walked through the unit of kids—from babies and toddlers to teen-
agers—lying behind their glass doors. They were all hooked up to intravenous lines as monitoring devices tracked their vital signs, and ventilators
sustained those unable to breathe themselves. If you want to confront the
pain and hardships of hospital work, I can think of no better place to visit
than a PICU or neonatal units.

That day, I saw in one of the rooms a heart-transplant patient, a teen-age girl who smiled at me as I passed by with the charge nurse. In another room, a boy had barely begun to recover from the traumatic brain injury caused by a hit-and-run accident that had left him unconscious for a few days; as John, one of the speech therapists, evaluated him for "swallow-ing," his nurse gave him an IV antibiotic. A couple of hours after I arrived, a young girl experiencing an acute diabetic episode was admitted, and a ten-month-old baby (from a poor and broken family) lay in another room, fighting a severe generalized infection and a variety of other compromising conditions; he had been a "code blue" during the night shift and had had to be resuscitated. Even though this was just "another day in the PICU," I could not help but wonder how everyone working there coped with it all, day in and day out for years—closely monitoring patients and getting them what they needed on time, putting on a good face for the distraught fami-lies, and maintaining an even keel in an atmosphere where life and death hang in the balance.

During this visit, there had been a lot of commotion as one of the attend-ing physicians, the charge nurse, the bedside nurse, and the social worker actively talked to a patient's parents about the condition of their child. The seven-week-old baby had been initially diagnosed with sudden infant death syndrome (SIDS), but after some investigating, the health-care staff learned that the mother had fallen asleep on him while breastfeeding and acciden-tally asphixiated him. Even though he had been resuscitated several times and kept alive for a few days, many neurological tests had confirmed ir-reversible brain damage. The health-care team had finally agreed that there was no possibility of recovery whatsoever, and in a "family conference" they informed the baby's parents that they had to consider removing him from the machines that were keeping his body functioning. "He will never wake up," the attending physician said, in a grave and soft tone.

While I was obviously moved by the sadness and pain of the situation, I was also trying to focus on how the practitioners were handling the dif-ficult circumstance and working with each other (even though my project truly seemed such a superficial enterprise, given what I was witnessing—an occasion in which professionalism and caring were united, but at the end of a life). Jaime, the nurse, who was caring for this baby (and his family) and another patient in the next room, would do everything she needed to do for both of them. Martha, the social worker, stayed vigilant at the parents' side, talking to them and trying to give them comfort as they cried. Dr. Wilkinson never left the unit: he checked on the patient regularly and answered every question from the parents, even when they had asked the same question a few minutes earlier. The respiratory therapist, Mike, was in the room frequently, checking the ventilator and talking to the nurse and the physician. Everyone seemed emotionally affected but on task; after all, "this is our job," Jaime told me, as she prepared a syringe with medication for her other patient.

As the day progressed, the baby's family painfully decided to "let him go," and Jaime devoted her attention to how things would proceed. Physician, nurse, social worker, and respiratory therapist were there as more family members (siblings, grandparents, aunts, uncles, and cousins) arrived and everyone gathered around the child. Jaime closed all the blinds, the curtains, and the heavy sliding glass door to give the family privacy.

I felt sick to my stomach, anticipating what would happen in the minutes ahead. Then, everything seemed to stand still and I felt an overwhelming silence. When the family was ready to let go, they all held hands, the mother held her baby, and Dr. Wilkinson turned off the machines. Jaime put her hand on the mother's shoulder as Martha put hers on the father's shoulder. Dr. Wilkinson remained composed without saying anything, as did Mike, who stood in a corner of the room. After a few minutes, the physician expressed his condolences, awkwardly returning a hug from the baby's mother and shaking the father's hand. Martha stayed with them and reassured them that everything would be all right. Jaime hugged the parents and left the room crying, her pager beeping incessantly (it was her other patient calling). Mike expressed his condolences and left to check on his other patients.

I left the hospital that day shaken and deeply saddened, but the experience underscored for me the balancing act of practitioners in Hospital General. Beyond the obvious "life lessons" of such dire circumstances, this episode illustrates how professionalism and caring are not merely analytical categories to be deconstructed and cross-examined. Rather, they reveal a great deal about our social reality: what matters to us, why work is meaningful, and the values we embrace, protect, and wish to pass on.

Notes

Introduction

1. Derber, "Toward a New Theory"; and Hartley, "System of Alignments."
2. Nonetheless, occupational status scales still rank "physician" as one of the most highly prestigious occupations, followed closely by "registered nurse." See, for example, Nam and Boyd, "Occupational Status in 2000."
3. The systematic accounts include Allen, *Changing Shape*; Becker et al., *Boys in White*; Brannon, *Intensifying Care*; Brodkin Sacks, *Caring by the Hour*; Freidson, *Hospital in Modern Society*; Goodman-Draper, *Health Care's Forgotten Majority*; Strauss et al., "Hospital"; and Sweet, *God's Hotel*. For the organizational point of view, see Starr, *Social Transformation*; Griffin, *Hospitals*; Salamon, *Hospital*; and Makary, *Unaccountable*.
4. "Hospital General" is a pseudonym, as are the names of all the people whom I interviewed. Many of the events and some of the descriptors of people I interviewed have been altered enough to maintain anonymity without undermining their analytical value.
5. For two important exceptions, see Abbott and Meerabeau, *Sociology*, and Chambliss, *Beyond Caring*. Studies of nursing home work have also focused attention on the professional-care relationship, especially Foner, *Caregiving Dilemma*, and C. L. Stacey, *Caring Self*. See also Zussman, *Intensive Care*, for a more critical assessment of the caring-professional relationship, and Sweet, *God's Hotel*, for an intimate account of preserving the caring ideal in the face of contrary trends in medicine.
6. See under "Reports" at the Institute of Medicine website (*www.iom.edu*), and especially *The Future of Nursing: Leading Change, Advancing Health*, which states that "nurses should be full partners, with physicians and other health care professionals, in redesigning health care in the United States" (1).
7. Wright, "Francis Report." "The most basic standards of care were not observed," noted Francis, "and fundamental rights to dignity were not respected" (quoted in Wright). For complete documentation of the Francis report, see the website of the Mid Staffordshire NHS Foundation Trust Public Inquiry, *midstaffspublicinquiry.com*.
8. Goffman, *Asylums*; and Caudill, *Psychiatric Hospital*. See also Wallace, *Total Institutions*.
9. Strauss, *Negotiations*; Strauss, *Medical Ghettos*; Strauss, *Psychiatric Ideologies and Institutions*; and Strauss et al., *Social Organization*. For more recent applica-

tions of this approach, see Allen, "Narrating Nursing Jurisdiction"; Allen, "Doing Occupational Demarcation"; and Allen, "Nursing-Medical Boundary."

10. Strauss et al., "Hospital," 154.

11. Ibid., 156.

12. Abbott, "Things of Boundaries"; and Abbott, *System of Professions*.

13. Finn et al., "Some Unintended Effects"; and Finn, "Language of Teamwork." See also Dingwall, "Problems of Teamwork."

14. On family, see Jacobs and Gerson, *Time Divide*. On schools, see Noddings, *Challenge to Care*, and Noddings, *Caring*. On the workplace in general, see Hochschild, *Managed Heart*. Regarding health care in particular, feminist scholars can be credited for reexamining professionalism and its principles of objectivity, detachment, and rational, deductive principles based on scientific norms. For example, see Graham, "Caring"; M. Stacey, "Division of Labour Revisited"; Ungerson, *Gender and Caring*; Ungerson, "Why Do Women Care"; Waerness, "Rationality of Caring"; and Witz, *Professions and Patriarchy*. Celia Davies, in "Competence versus Care," notes that conceptualizations of professions and medicine are embedded in "a notion of scientific rationality, [which] denied a place for emotions and . . . this restricted the very definition of [professional] work" (23). She asserts that caring has been ignored or devalued as women's "natural" inclination and has remained under-theorized and inadequately conceptualized; caring is hard to measure or quantify and the practice of professional care in medicine is difficult to put into words. Davies contends that social scientists must recognize the social processes that have denied caring an equal footing with medical work. In order to do this, one must examine "the cultural content of gender, specifically . . . the *metaphors of masculinity* that give a sense of vision and purpose to the public world [. . .] and inform the notions of bureaucracy and profession" (23). Feminist critics suggest that caring, whether the caregiving takes place in the home or in the hospital, is intrinsically different from curing and contradictory to masculine values espoused in the professions. Caring presupposes femininity; it is affective, relational, and expressive. For example, Arlene Kaplan Daniels in "Invisible Work" argues that there is an undeniable link between caregiving in the home and paid care work; that is, the more the activities of paid care such as nursing (and arguably other professions) resemble the nurturing activities of domestic work, the more they are seen as womanly. Undoubtedly, the care work model highlights not only the centrality of gender processes in the workplace but also the importance of care work in understanding the relative subordination of semi-professions vis-à-vis classic professions. However, it fails to fully develop the notion of caring as an ideology and a set of occasionally contested practices constituting the work of professionals and semi-professionals alike, particularly in medical and health care settings. For a recent overview of the definition, measurement, and valuation of care work, the problems associated with the gendered nature of care provision, and the social policy implications in resolving issue, see Folbre, *For Love and Money*.

15. See Apesoa-Varano, "Educated Caring," regarding the students I interviewed.
16. Allen, "Re-reading Nursing," 280.
17. Nelson and Gordon, *Complexities of Care*, 13–29.
18. Anspach, *Deciding Who Lives*, 80.
19. Steven H. Lopez, in "Emotional Labor," makes a useful distinction between emotional labor, which he argues is coerced via organizations and is therefore an alienated and exploited form of labor, and organized emotional care, in which organizations provide structural support for autonomous self-directed caregiving as an important and valued aspect of many jobs, including but not limited to professional work.
20. For an example of how caring constitutes resistance to bureaucratic forms of control, see Foner's insightful analysis in *Caregiving Dilemma*, 131–38. See also Lopez, "Emotional Labor," for a more optimistic view of emotive caring as a beneficial feature of organizational settings.
21. For a useful and precise discussion of the meanings and role of the term ideology, a good starting point would be Bennett Berger's *Essay on Culture*.
22. Though I interviewed nearly half of all the OPS therapists, respiratory therapists, and social workers, my sample of physicians and nurses is not representative by any means. Nonetheless, I sought to interview as many physicians and nurses of various specialties and on different units as I could.
23. Two notable exceptions to the focus on physician-nurse and professional-client relationships are Finn, "Language of Teamwork," and Dingwall, "Problems of Teamwork."
24. Important to debates about professions—what they are, who belongs, the criteria for inclusion and exclusion and so forth—have been parallel debates about related occupations that have been deemed not "truly" professional; that is, semi-professions such as nursing, social work, librarianship, and teaching. Amitai Etzioni, in *The Semi-Professions and Their Organization*, exemplified this perspective by arguing that practitioners of nursing, social work, and teaching (among other occupations) could not be considered "true" professionals because they lacked extensive specialized knowledge and had little autonomy and control over their work. He also pointed out that the semi-professions' subordinate status could be explained partly in terms of their gender composition, with women as opposed to men carrying out what was considered non-technical, less skilled work. Although sensitive to the issue of gender, Etzioni failed to see these occupations in a dynamic or contextually specific way and the 'semi-profession as a degraded profession' perspective is thus limited in several ways. Aside from the fact that the lower value that Etzioni attached to semi-professional work reflected gender biases about the nature of the work itself, many semi-professional fields, such as nursing, social work, and therapists, require higher education, licensing, and enjoy more autonomy and control today than might be imagined from this perspective. Neither their training nor their experiences are as simplified or unskilled as portrayed in earlier literature. And even if social scientists

theoretically considered nurses, social workers, paralegals and others to be semi-professionals—not "true" professionals—these employees themselves often deeply identify as professionals, experience themselves as professional workers, and present themselves as professionals to others.

Chapter 1

1. See Larson, *Rise of Professionalism*; Freidson, *Profession of Medicine*; and Freidson, *Professional Dominance*. This autonomy extends beyond the workplace to include the reproduction of occupational members through recruitment and training at university and postgraduate institutions.

2. In 2005, Hospital General offered over forty-two medical specialties, with a total of approximately 5,000 full-time staff working in the hospital, including approximately 500 attending/faculty physicians, 700 residents and fellows, 1,200 registered nurses (1,000 women, 200 men), 40 occupational, physical, and speech therapists (30 women, 10 men), 40 social workers (37 women, 3 men), and 50 respiratory therapists (28 women, 22 men), as well as (this is not an exhaustive list) clerical and administrative personnel, registered pharmacists, registered nutritionists, radiology technicians, laboratory technicians, medical interpreters, volunteers, chaplains, and food, janitorial, transport, and ground maintenance workers. According to public disclosures, the hospital's operating budget was approximately $800 million, with externally funding for medical research exceeding $100 million. That same year, the hospital reported having approximately fifty general and specialist units, eight intensive care units, and more than fifteen operating rooms. It held 577 licensed acute-care beds, with an average daily inpatient census of 425 and an average length of inpatient stay of 4.7 days. The hospital records showed an annual average of approximately 46,196 emergency room visits, 32,886 inpatient admissions, and 863,394 outpatient clinic visits.

3. Finn, "Language of Teamwork," 104; and Finn et al., "Some Unintended Effects," 1150.

4. I emphasize *some* status, respect, and ideological leverage, because one must recognize that historically the subordinate position of nurses has also been linked to their embrace of caring. See, for example, Chambliss, *Beyond Caring*; Nelson and Gordon, *Complexities of Care*; D'Antonio, *American Nursing*; Melosh, *Physician's Hand*; and Reverby, *Ordered to Care*. But see also Dingwall and Allen, "Implications of Healthcare Reforms," and Davina Allen's compelling critique of this strategy in nursing, "Re-reading Nursing."

5. See Rodwin, *Conflicts of Interest*; Rodwin, *Medicine, Money, and Morals*; Gawande, *Better*; Groopman, *How Doctors Think*; Gruen et al., "Public Roles"; Hafferty, "Professionalism"; Royal College of Physicians, *Doctors in Society*; Light, "Countervailing Power"; Wolinsky, "Professional Dominance"; and Wailoo et al., "Professional Sovereignty."

6. Rodwin, *Medicine, Money, and Morals*.

7. Starr, *Social Transformation*, 393. Starr notes that "this ambivalence is evident in the patients' rights and women's movements [of the 1970s], which simultaneously claimed rights of access to and rights of protection against medical authority" (393). While this public disenchantment centered on physician authority, Starr notes that increasing medical costs and physician fees also raised the public's ire as the adoption of fixed fee schedules through the hospital-Medicare-Medicaid nexus led to "rampant inflation in medical fees" (385). See also Campbell et al., "National Survey"; and Rodwin, *Conflicts of Interest*.

8. Wolinsky and Brune, *Serpent on the Staff*.

9. Freidson, *Professionalism*.

10. As Atul Gawande, a surgeon at Brigham and Women's Hospital in Boston and an associate professor at Harvard Medical School, notes in "Personal Best" (46), "Knowledge of disease and the science of treatment are always evolving. We have to keep developing our capabilities and avoid falling behind. So the training inculcates an ethic of perfectionism. Expertise is thought to be not a static condition but one that doctors must build and sustain *for themselves*" (emphasis added). Gawande argues that doctors, and in his case specifically surgeons, would benefit from using coaches to help them improve their techniques like professionals in the fields of sports, the arts, or teaching. Yet as my interviews show, and Gawande acknowledges, this is alien to the individualized professional self of physicians.

11. Halpern, "Dynamics of Professional Control."

12. Peters, *Powerful Occupational Therapists*.

13. Moffat, "History of Physical Therapy."

14. Wallis, "Profession and Professionalism" (parts 1 and 2); and Cusick and Adamson, "Professional Accreditation."

15. Granted, this may not hold for OPS therapists who either practice independently or work in smaller clinics without physicians.

16. Muff, *Socialization, Sexism, and Stereotyping*; and Neil and Watts, *Caring and Nursing*.

17. L. A. Jacobs et al., "Baccalaureate Degree in Nursing"; Melia, *Learning and Working*; Melia, "Student Nurses' Construction"; Melosh, *Physician's Hand*; Melosh, "Not Merely a Profession"; Reverby, *Ordered to Care*; J. Williams, "What Is a Profession"; and C. L. Williams, *Still a Man's World*. See also D'Antonio, *American Nursing*.

18. Cohen, *Nurse's Quest*; and Melosh, *Physician's Hand*.

19. Nelson and Gordon, *Complexities of Care*, 1–29, 104–21.

20. Anspach documents this characteristic in *Deciding Who Lives*.

21. This tension is understandable in the context of Nelson and Gordon's argument that traditional images of nursing still haunt an occupation struggling for a more respected future. See also Dingwall and Allen, "Implications of Healthcare Reforms."

22. Allen, "Re-reading Nursing."

23. Held, *Ethics of Care*; and Apesoa-Varano, "Educated Caring."

24. Apesoa-Varano, "Educated Caring."

25. Larkin, "Medical Dominance and Control"; and K. J. Stewart, "Promoting Professionalism." Radiology technician is another occupation that similarly lacks autonomy.

26. Mishoe, "Current and Future Credentialing"; Shelledy and Wiezalis, "Education and Credentialing"; and K. J. Stewart, "Promoting Professionalism." The skepticism over increased credentialing voiced by RTs should not be construed as a sign of their being antiknowledge.

27. In relation to psychiatry, see Abbott, *System of Professions*; Walkowitz, *Working with Class*; Sibeon, "Construction"; and Sibeon, "Social Work Knowledge." See also Etzioni, *Semi-Professions and Their Organization*.

28. Crocker, *Social Work*; Ehrenreich, *Altruistic Imagination*; Etzioni, *Semi-Professions and Their Organization*; Haynes, "Rank and File Movement"; Kunzel, *Fallen Women, Problem Girls*; Leiby, *History of Social Welfare*; Leighninger, *Social Work*; Spano, *Rank and File Movement*; and Wenocur and Reisch, *From Charity to Enterprise*.

29. Beckett and Maynard, *Values and Ethics*.

30. See Hugman, "Social Work and De-professionalization," but see also Beder, *Hospital Social Work*.

31. The importance of knowledge as *the* major axis of status conflicts—even for those ranked "below" the practitioners I spoke with—was reinforced for me as I read a student's paper while completing this book. In it, she wrote, "Within the hospital (another within the region) my position (patient 'transporter' in the radiology department) has very little status and many workers that occupy the higher status positions such as x-ray techs, nurses, and respiratory therapists often treat people in my position with disrespect by yelling at us and ignoring us when we cross paths within the hallways. However I've noticed that after I introduce myself and tell them that I'm going to school at university, they began to treat me with more respect. Instead of ignoring me in the hallway, one might ask 'how is school going?' I feel as though once they find out that I'm going to school that it raises my personal status and provides for more respect within the hospital institution." Apparently, even for those practitioners I consider who are ranked lower in the status hierarchy of knowledge, there is always someone lower. (Quotation included with permission of the student.)

32. As Finn et al. note in "Some Unintended Effects" (1149), teamwork "reproduces and maintains various forms of occupational inequality, as well as obscuring the need for more fundamental changes in the work and social context, both from the perspective of those who wish to reform healthcare and of those who would wish to see a more equitable workplace." As will become clear in the next chapter, I agree with this appraisal and would add that teamwork also obscures the organizational neglect of caring.

Chapter 2

1. See Varano, *Forced Choices*; Russell, *Sharing Ownership*; and Parker and Slaughter, *Choosing Sides*. For an example of this in a white-collar bank setting, see Smith, *Managing*.

2. Rachael Finn, in "Language of Teamwork," adopts a similar approach in her work on teamwork in the medical setting. Finn writes that teamwork exists not as "an empirical reality," but as a social construction "and a discursive resource through which particular interest-based versions of reality are constituted" (104). Finn distinguishes "*team work* as material practice" from "*teamwork* as discourse," and focuses on "the ideological uses and effects of *teamwork* within the distinct set of social structures characterizing the medical division of labour" (ibid.).

3. Abbott, *System of Professions*.

4. Finn et al., "Some Unintended Effects," 1149. Finn and her colleagues further note that "the form that teamwork takes in any given context, therefore, is the outcome of these micro-political struggles. While the collaborative teamwork ideology is a potential form of social control, promoting cooperation and preventing conflict among disparate professionals . . . , its inherent ambiguity as a 'loose rubric for action' opens space for the negotiation of working arrangements in the context of established authority relationships" (1149).

5. My ethnography of teamwork richly illustrates Magali Sarfatti Larson's argument of how occupations must forge their special (professional) status within organizational bureaucracies composed of other occupations competing for such status. She focuses on engineering as the typical case of professionalism in contemporary organizations, whereas my study documents this process among medical workers in the hospital setting. See also Finn, "Language of Teamwork"; Finn et al., "Some Unintended Effects"; and Garman et al., "Worldviews in Collision."

6. This was also frequently true of nurses, who needed to reaffirm their professional self.

7. For some exceptions to the rule, though, one might begin with Shoshana Zuboff's *In the Age of the Smart Machine*, which considers the negative impact of computer technology on occupations such as accounting, finance, insurance, and technology industries.

8. See Allen, "Re-reading Nursing," for an argument of the strategic importance of this coordinator role in advancing the nursing profession.

9. As Finn et al. note of medical records clerks, "below a certain level in the organization, one does not qualify for team membership at all; therefore one cannot plausibly use a teamwork discourse to advance claims to equality" ("Some Unintended Effects," 1152). The case of respiratory technicians differs insofar as they work with patients, and at Hospital General they frequently challenged other practitioners (including physicians), but not always with success.

10. See, for example, deLamerens-Pratt and Golden, "Teamwork in Medical Settings."

11. While the research findings of Finn et al. lead them to reject what they consider the "more dystopian visions of managerial control" through teamwork ("Some

Unintended Effects," 1153), another study by Finn ("Language of Teamwork," 123) and my data still point to the role of a teamwork ideology in obscuring how control is wielded and redirecting attention away from organizational/structural factors to occupational/personality factors as responsible for conflicts between practitioners.

12. For example, in a letter to the editor of the *New Yorker* (October 24, 2011, 3), Virginia Tyack commented on an article by surgeon Atul Gawande ("Personal Best"), who argued on behalf of surgeons having coaches so as to improve their skills and procedures. Tyack wrote, "I once worked in a lowly position in an operating room. I was never consulted about how any aspect of a procedure, however minor, might be improved, until the hospital was faced with a malpractice lawsuit. Suddenly, it seemed, the surgeon, the hospital administrator, and the lawyers were interested in my intimate knowledge of that particular case and what I thought might have gone wrong. Perhaps another approach to improving patient outcomes might be routine 'post-game' reviews with the entire surgical team. Good outcomes, after all, depend on the continuing development of everyone involved."

13. The wax and wane of physician power has been well documented by Starr, Larson, Freidson, and Light, among others, but Finn is less convinced that the teamwork ideal may engender calls for more egalitarian changes in the healthcare division of labor. Writing of the British context and National Health Service, Finn notes: "While statements of policy aspirations emphasizing the breaking down of professional hierarchies, joint effort and shared responsibility opens up space for the negotiation of egalitarian working, its ambiguity does not present a challenge to social structures from which nurses and ODPs [Operating Department Practitioners] could speak from legitimately with voice. This is politically functional, as a means of sustaining the input of nurses and ODPs and achieving efficient, safe outcomes without the need for increased material reward or radical systemic change" ("Language of Teamwork," 126). See also Garman et al., "Worldviews in Collision."

Chapter 3

1. See Allen, "Re-reading Nursing"; Dingwall and Allen, "Implications of Healthcare Reforms"; and Nelson and Gordon, *Complexities of Care.*

2. Friedman, "Beyond Caring"; Harrington Meyer, *Care Work*; Ungerson, *Gender and Caring*; and Waerness, "Rationality of Caring."

3. This may not be the case with primary care physicians in outpatient clinics, though, as Apesoa-Varano et al. note in "Curing and Caring."

4. Groopman, *How Doctors Think*; Di Blasi et al., "Influence of Context Effects"; Kaplan et al., "Assessing the Effects"; M. A. Stewart, "Effective Physician-Patient Communication"; Agency for Healthcare Research and Quality, *National Healthcare Disparities Report*; Cheung et al., "Nursing Care"; and M. A. Stewart et al., "Impact of Patient-Centered Care." See also Larson and Yao, "Clinical Empathy,"

and Brooten and Naylor, "Nurses' Effect."

5. On medical school trends, see Patterson et al., "Effecting." A memo sent to all medical and resident medical staff provided an example of institutional pressure.

6. See Allen, "Re-reading Nursing," 274–75, for how much nurses are required to circulate and integrate individuals into the healthcare organization while mitigating its most dehumanizing aspects.

7. Also, the type and objective of the nurses' interventions were fundamentally directed at alleviating short-term physical issues. This is somewhat consistent with Nelson and Gordon's argument (in *Complexities of Care*) that nursing discourse neglects the long-term diagnostic and interventionist role nurses play in patient well-being and ultimate recovery. But see also Wicks's account of Australian nurses and their contradictory discourses on nursing in *Nurses and Doctors*.

8. See C. Davies, *Gender*; C. Davies, "New Vision of Professionalism"; and Salvage, "Rethinking Professionalism." While social workers are most able to perform emotive caring for the same reasons as OPS therapists, they are distinct in one way: they had fewer opportunities for circumventing, neglecting, or dismissing caring compared with the other groups whose work centered on physical treatment. For social workers, emotive caring definitely fell under their professional jurisdiction. Even when confronting unfavorable working conditions such as lack of time, understaffing, or emotional burnout, social workers had no choice but to fulfill this dimension of their work role. Having said all this, I am not arguing that all OPS therapists and social workers performed caring or that these two groups always did caring work. Likewise, I am not suggesting that physicians, nurses, and RTs never did, for there are always individual exceptions and circumstances to the contrary. Rather, I am noting that some occupational groups are more likely than others to perform emotive caring for reasons beyond the individual; that is, reasons related to the various labor processes in the hospital, prevalent expectations about these groups' caring roles, the groups' professional ideology, and existing working conditions.

9. Leiby, *History of Social Welfare*; and Walkowitz, *Working with Class*.

10. For scholarship on caring, see Bowden, *Caring*; Harrington Meyer, *Care Work*; Held, *Ethics of Care*; and Ungerson, *Gender and Caring*. On the new professionalism, see C. Davies, *Gender*; Salvage, "Rethinking Professionalism"; and Hugman, *New Approaches*. An interesting and very telling interpretation of the "hand-holding" metaphor used repeatedly by all the practitioners I spoke with is how emotive caring can be seen as an infantilizing of patients (as voiced in this chapter's epigraph). Unfortunately, this not only further diminishes the importance of emotive caring for both patient and practitioner well-being, it also perpetuates the expert-patient asymmetry characteristic of the hospital context and is the antipathy of the new professionalism espoused by Davies, Salvage, and Hugman.

Chapter 4

1. Unfortunately, because of hospital policy and confidentiality issues, I am unable to discuss these in more detail or cite the publication as a source.
2. Hochschild, *Managed Heart*.
3. On the topic of exploitation, see Leidner, "Serving Hamburgers"; C. L. Stacey, "Labor's Love Learned"; and Foner, *Caregiving Dilemma*.
4. For example, Glomb et al., in "Emotional Labor Demands," find that emotional labor is rewarded for jobs requiring more cognitive demands, while jobs with fewer cognitive demands suffer a wage penalty. This does not mean, as I have argued, that practitioners who expend emotional labor do not deploy complex knowledge or skills in their jobs; it is only less compared to physicians *as the status hierarchy is conceived*. As England et al. (in "Wages of Virtue") and Reskin and Roos (in *Job Queues, Gender Queues*) have argued, this wage differential is due to the gendering of skill sets associated with emotional labor.
5. Chambliss, *Beyond Caring*, 68. Also see C. Davies, *Gender*; C. Davies, "Competence versus Care?"; Foner, *Caregiving Dilemma*; Tronto, "Care"; and Tronto, *Moral Boundaries*.
6. Goffman, *Asylums*, 4−5.
7. For a related analysis of how a large corporation institutionalizes a new ideology and seeks to reinforce it via workshop training, see Vicki Smith, *Managing*, 54−86.
8. "Future Care Incorporated" is a pseudonym. I attended the workshop in its entirety and participated in all its activities.
9. Ducey, *Never Good Enough*, 15.
10. Ibid., 112.
11. See Berger, *Essay on Culture*. And as Ariel Ducey documents in the training sessions she observed, not only did participants routinely challenge the ideological precepts of the training programs and instruction they received, but many were actually emboldened to speak out to and against hospital management (*Never Good Enough*, 139−58).
12. See Allen, "Re-reading Nursing," 273−74.
13. Examples of resistance include workers not showing up for work or "working to rule," and students "ditching" or being inattentive in class. Likewise, song, humor, dance, or even silent prayer can constitute meaningful forms of resistance to oppression or injustice. Rick Fantasia makes this case for nurses in *Cultures of Solidarity*, 121−79. See also Hodson, "Worker Resistance."
14. Lopez, "Emotional Labor."
15. On nurses harboring the myth, see Nelson and Gordon, *Complexities of Care*, and Dingwall and Allen, "Implications of Healthcare Reforms."

Chapter 5

1. Goldsmith, *Can Hospitals Survive*; Martin, *Hospitals in Trouble*; Strauss et al., *Social Organization*; Weinberg, *Code Green*; Wilkerson, "Political Economy of

Health"; and Wolinsky, "Professional Dominance."

2.   Barlett and Steele, "Critical Condition"; Bazzoli, "Corporatization of American Hospitals"; Derber, "Toward a New Theory"; Campbell et al., "National Survey"; Hafferty and Light, "Professional Dynamics"; Zugar, "Dissatisfaction with Medical Practice"; and McKinlay and Marceau, "End."

3.   Luepke, "White Coat, Blue Collar"; Albert, "More Doctors Following Trend"; Budrys, *When Physicians Join Unions*; Choudhry and Brennan, "Collective Bargaining by Physicians"; and Hoff, "Physician Unionization."

4.   Ducey, *Never Good Enough*, 3; Diamond, *Making Gray Gold*; Goodman-Draper, *Health Care's Forgotten Majority*; and Foner, *Caregiving Dilemma*.

5.   Thomas and Thomas, *Child in America*, 572.

6.   A listing of these trenchant ethnographies is beyond the scope of this book, but one could start at no better place than Barbara Garson's *All the Livelong Day*.

7.   See Shanafelt et al., "Burnout and Satisfaction," which reported that burnout was more common among physicians, especially specialists, than among other U.S. workers.

8.   Referencing the 2004 edition of the widely cited national survey of nurses, *The Registered Nurse Population* (tables 40 and 33), D'Antonio notes that "respondents that left nursing reported that they did so because of stressful work environments, long hours, and low salaries. Still, 76 percent of those nurses who remained, and 74 percent of those working in the most direct and intense hospital staff nursing roles, also described themselves as moderately or extremely satisfied with their positions" (*American Nursing*, 180). In Health Resources and Services Administration, *The Registered Nurse Population: Findings from the 2008 National Sample Survey of Registered Nurses*, the updated percentages are similar.

9.   For a related analysis, see Allen, "Doctor-Nurse Relationships."

10. See Reverby, *Ordered to Care*; and D'Antonio, *American Nursing*.

11. This cost has also been noted by many scholars of social work. See Abbott and Meerabeau, *Sociology*; Hugman, *New Approaches*; MacCallum, "Case in Social Work"; Sibeon, "Social Work Knowledge"; and Walkowitz, *Working with Class*.

12. Budd and Sharma, *Healing Bond*; C. Davies, "Competence versus Care?"; Dorroh, *Between Patient*; Emerick, *Client-Clinician Relationship*; Friedman and DiMatteo, *Interpersonal Issues*; Heritage and Maynard, *Communication in Medical Care*; Hinz, *Communicating with Patients*; Myerscough and Ford, *Talking with Patients*; and Van Servellen, *Communication Skills*.

13. Beauchamp and Childress, *Principles of Biomedical Ethics*; Fagerhaugh and Strauss, *Politics of Pain Management*; Surbone and Zwitter, *Communication*; and Budd and Sharma, *Healing Bond*.

14. Hurwitz et al., *Narrative Research*.

15. See Mechanic, *Mental Health*; Mechanic, *Truth about Health Care*; Light and Levine, "Changing Character"; Freidson, *Professionalism*; and Starr, *Social Transformation*.

16. Kemp, *Mental Health in America*; Howard and Strauss, *Humanizing Health Care*; Wallace, *Total Institutions*; Caudill, *Psychiatric Hospital*; and Goffman, *Asylums*.

17. Bowers, *Interpersonal Relationships*; and Lipkin and Cohen, *Effective Approaches*.

18. For related discussions, see Braithwaite and Japp, "They Make Us Miserable"; Ford and Christmon, "Every Breast Cancer"; Rintamaki and Brashers, "Social Identity"; and Thompson and Gilloti, "Staying Out."

19. DiMatteo and DiNicola, *Achieving Patient Compliance*; and Lorber, "Good Patients, Problem Patients."

20. I could not, however, confirm this estimate.

21. For the issue of cultural competency in medical care, see Angelelli and Geist-Martin, "Enhancing," and Lo and Stacey, "Beyond Cultural Competency."

22. Bishop and Scudder, *Caring, Curing, Coping*; and Fagerhaugh and Strauss, *Politics of Pain Management*.

23. Leander et al., *Patients First*.

24. DiMatteo and DiNicola, *Achieving Patient Compliance*; and Hurwitz et al., *Narrative Research*.

25. Clair and Allman, *Sociomedical Perspectives*; and Peabody, *Doctor and Patient*. For a related argument about science, see Keller, *Making Sense of Life*, and Keller and Longino, *Feminism and Science*.

26. It is possible, however, that such awkward interactions were not as frequent or severe as described by the RTs, because the condition of the patients they most often treated casts some doubt on their claims. A significant number of RTs work with patients who are unable to interact or talk because they are, for example, on ventilators or sedated. Likewise, as I have noted, the RTs' work was mostly technical and involved dealing more directly with medical equipment than patients per se. Consequently, compared to other bedside practitioners, they may in fact face fewer conflicts, but those they do encounter stand out, given their infrequent verbal exchanges with patients.

27. For related discussions in other contexts, see Gans, *War against the Poor*; Gans, *Urban Villagers*; Liebow, *Tally's Corner*; Liebow, *Tell Them*; and Kunzel, *Fallen Women, Problem Girls*.

28. Once again, this is not to say that the practitioners found interacting with patients professionally or emotionally unrewarding, but I note how frequently they *considered* it a problem (as do teachers regarding student interaction, at all levels of schooling, even as they too find professional and emotional fulfillment in their work). This could be a matter of high expectations courting deep frustrations.

29. Allsop and Saks, *Regulating the Health Professions*; McMurtry, *Hospital Nursing*; Choi et al., *Governing University Hospitals*; and Weinberg, *Code Green*.

30. Goldsmith, *Can Hospitals Survive*; Hollingsworth and Hollingsworth, *Controversy about American Hospitals*; and Martin, *Hospitals in Trouble*.

31. For similar findings, see Schuhmann, "Hospital Financial Performance Trends." For privacy and ethical considerations, I have refrained from fully disclosing the official reports I obtained about the hospital's annual financial statements and

related information. I was able to obtain similar information from public records about other hospitals in the area.

32. See Larson, *Rise of Professionalism*, and Starr, *Social Transformation*, but also Ehrenreich and Ehrenreich, "Professional-Managerial Class," and Gouldner, *Future of Intellectuals*.

33. A conflicted class of managers may be more appropriate if one considers practitioners and hospital management as members of an otherwise unified professional-managerial class, as the Ehrenreichs argue ("Professional-Managerial Class").

34. My point here differs from Rachael Finn's compelling argument in "Language of Teamwork" (123), which asserts that by casting problems and their solution in terms of individual professional members, practitioners "create individualized constructions, such that wider organizational and social structural factors are not constituted as significant." I am arguing that in this context it is the practitioners' *collective conscience* against management that paradoxically obscures the occupational hierarchy and impedes collective mobilization against their managerial counterparts.

Chapter 6

1. See also Freidson, *Profession of Medicine*; Freidson, *Professional Dominance*; Hafferty, "Professionalism"; Haskell, *Authority of Experts*; Kimball, *True Professional Ideal*; and Lively, "Occupational Claims to Professionalism."

2. On ethnicity and race, see Cornell and Hartmann, *Ethnicity and Race*. On gender and sexuality, see Thorne, *Gender Play*; Epstein, *Deceptive Distinctions*; Epstein, "Tinkerbells and Pinups"; and Gerson and Peiss, "Boundaries, Negotiations, Consciousness." On class, see Lamont, *Money, Morals, and Manners*. On the professions and work, see Lamont and Molnar, "Study of Boundaries."

3. Epstein, "Tinkerbells and Pinups," 233. Though boundaries may be structural, say, for instance in the labor and housing markets, or postgraduate recruitment and matriculation, they are also symbolic and may thus linger on well after structural boundaries have changed. "Attitudes may remain independent of behavior," Epstein writes (234). "After all, individuals and groups develop investments in boundary distinctions. For individuals, boundaries define who they think they are." The conceptual distinctions or symbolic criteria used to mark off boundaries can take many forms and though they may overlap or exist along a continuum, they are most frequently understood in dichotomous terms, such as black/white, rich/poor, and male/female. And while these criteria commonly elicit consensus, as conceptual markers they can often be ambiguous or disputed by people on opposite sides of the boundary or even within the same side. Central to such self-definitions is one's position vis-à-vis others in structured hierarchies of inequality and domination. Research on boundaries has been concerned with how various social inequalities are constructed and reproduced. Epstein (236) notes, "As individuals have interests in the material conditions of their lives and fight to

maintain their advantages and their territory, they also have an interest in preserving their identities. As we shall see, some of the reasons that people become invested in boundaries are because their sense of self, their security, their dignity, all are tied to particular boundary distinctions, and these personal investments are bound up with authority and hierarchy."

4. For a classic analysis of how consent to exploitative labor relations is generated see Burawoy, *Manufacturing Consent*. Though my analysis of this process is similar, it transcends the larger context of capitalist relations of production, as it likely manifests in national health care systems as well.

5. Freidson, *Profession of Medicine*; for a related argument, see Gieryn, "Boundary Work."

6. For example, see Harvey's analysis of the "extended role" of intensive care nursing and midwifery in "Up-Skilling." For discussions that highlight the boundary conflicts revolving around the spheres of practice and authority that shape occupational hierarchy and professional prestige, see Timmons and Tanner's "Disputed Occupational Boundary," which studies struggles between operating room nurses and an emerging "new" profession, that of Operating Department Practitioners (ODPs), in Britain; Ben-Sira and Szyf's "Status Inequality," which focuses on the ensuing boundary conflicts between nurses and social workers in an Israeli hospital" (but see also Aldridge, "Unlimited Liability"); and Norris's research on various treatment providers of musculo-skeletal problems in New Zealand, in "How 'We' Are Different." In the Straussian tradition (Strauss, *Psychiatric Ideologies and Institutions*; Strauss et al., "Hospital and Its Negotiated Order"), Davina Allen has studied the nurse-physician boundary through "atrocity stories," defining them as "dramatic or shocking events that may take on a legendary or apocryphal status in the oral culture of an occupational group" ("Narrating Nursing Jurisdiction," 76) and examining how they play a "dual boundary-work function—they construct a boundary between nursing and other occupations while simultaneously constituting the nursing group" (98). Also in the Straussian tradition, Foley and Faircloth, in "Medicine as Discursive Resource," examine the narratives of Florida midwives and how they utilized a biomedical discourse to both reinforce their distinction from and collaboration with doctors.

7. For example, Porter's study of power relations between doctors and nurses in a Northern Ireland hospital in "Participant Observation Study," Svensson's interviews of nurses in five Swedish hospitals in "Interplay," Hughes's participant observation of a general hospital in Britain in "When Nurse Knows Best," and Mesler's analysis of clinical pharmacists in two northeastern teaching hospitals in the United States in "Boundary Encroachment" all emphasize how boundary work constitutes a negotiated order whereby structures of power are more malleable and fluid than macro models depict.

8. See Anspach, *Deciding Who Lives*, for a compelling example of the distinction between the "objective" data relied on by physicians and the "subjective, interactional cues" that nurses use in judging a patient's condition.

9. Timmons and Tanner, "Disputed Occupational Boundary." See also Hughes, "When Nurse Knows Best," and Svensson, "Interplay."

10. In "Status Inequality," Ben-Sira and Szyf focus on the ensuing boundary conflicts between nurses and social workers in an Israeli hospital. They found an interesting paradox which essentially underscores a demarcation issue. While nurses and social workers believed in collaboration and agreed on the importance of psycho-social treatment to promote patients' recovery, they fundamentally disagreed on who ought to carry out this work. The disagreement rested upon who actually is competent and "has the authority to render that assistance" (371). Ben-Sira and Szyf established that nurses' dominance in the nurse-social worker relationship was evident in their provision of psycho-social assistance, their views regarding their professional jurisdiction over this function, their use of discretion to refer patients to social workers, and their concession that social workers fulfill "administrative functions" (i.e., arranging welfare assistance for patients after discharge). They argued that given the primary goal of the hospital to provide bio-medical services, the role of social workers as concerning only the "psycho-social" arena justified their subordination to nurses. For a related discussion emphasizing interprofessional conflicts, see Aldridge, "Unlimited Liability."

11. See, however, Timmons and Tanner, "Disputed Occupational Boundary," and Tanner and Timmons, "Backstage," for—exceptions to this finding.

12. On nurses as extensions of physicians, see Melosh, *Physician's Hand*, and Melosh, "Not Merely a Profession," but see also Porter, "Participant Observation Study"; Svensson, "Interplay"; and Hughes, "When Nurse Knows Best." On the issue of work intensification, see Brannon, *Intensifying Care*; Brannon, "Professionalization and Work Intensification"; and Harvey, "Up-Skilling."

13. This is the flip side of what Anselm Strauss termed "articulation work" in "Work and the Division of Labor" (8–9). See also Allen, "Re-reading Nursing," 273–74.

14. Gawande, *Better*; Groopman, *How Doctors Think*; Groopman, "Doctors and Patients"; and Groopman, *Second Opinions*.

15. Abbott, *System of Professions*; and Gieryn, "Boundary-Work and the Demarcation." The debate over evidence-based medicine has generated a significant literature, and the interested reader may find the following references useful: Ashcroft, "Current Epistemological Problems"; B. Davies, "Death"; Feinstein and Horwitz, "Problems"; Mitchell, "Evidence-Based Practice"; Mykhalovskiy and Weir, "Problem of Evidence-Based Medicine; Sackett et al., "Evidence Based Medicine"; and Timmermans and Mauck, "Promises and Pitfalls."

16. Beardwood, "Loosening of Professional Boundaries"; Abbott, *System of Professions*; Allen, *Changing Shape*; Allen, "Narrating Nursing Jurisdiction"; Brannon, *Intensifying Care*; and Brannon, "Professionalization and Work Intensification."

17. Ben-Sira and Szyf, "Status Inequality."

18. For a related argument, see Allen, *Changing Shape*.

19. For similar examples, see Porter, "Participant Observation Study"; Svensson, "Interplay"; Hughes, "When Nurse Knows Best."

20. This process is similar to what Erving Goffman called "studied non-observance," whereby participants in an interaction overlook or ignore others' inappropriate or incompetent acts in order to permit a successful completion of the interaction. Similarly, dismissing others' recommendations closely resembles what Robert Merton called "institutional evasion" whereby practical exigencies require groups to ignore or actively evade long-standing norms or rules that govern social relationships so as not to risk greater social disorder. See Goffman, *Interaction Ritual*, and Merton, *Social Theory*.
21. Manthey, *Practice of Primary Nursing*.
22. Abbott, *System of Professions*, 35–58.
23. Abbott, *System of Professions*.
24. This subtly underscores the contestable nature of rational-legal authority—in the Weberian sense—at the interactional level on a daily basis.
25. C. Davies, "Competence versus Care"; and Salvage, "Rethinking Professionalism."
26. Svensson, "Interplay."

Chapter 7

1. Hwang, "Ratio Roundup."
2. Moberg, "Nurses Fight."
3. Guadagnino, "Physician Unions Gain Steam"; Unland, "Physician Unions"; and Bazzoli, "Changes." See also Luepke, "White Coat, Blue Collar"; Albert, "More Doctors Following Trend"; Budrys, *When Physicians Join Unions*; Choudhry et al., "Collective Bargaining by Physicians"; and Hoff, "Physician Unionization."
4. Baumann and Silverman, "De-Professionalization in Health Care"; Saks, *Professions*; and Sullivan, "What Is Left."
5. Burkett and Kurz, "Comparison"; Department of Labor, "Gender Gap"; Schur and Kruse, "Gender Differences in Attitudes"; Riska, "Towards Gender Balance"; and Jacobs and Boulis, *Changing Face of Medicine*.
6. Fantasia, *Cultures of Solidarity*; Luepke, "White Coat, Blue Collar"; and Budrys, *When Physicians Join Unions*.
7. J. S. Finch, "Unionization in Respiratory Therapy."
8. De Tocqueville, *Democracy in America*.

Conclusion

1. Larson, *Rise of Professionalism*, 220.
2. On the relationship between emotive caring and successful outcomes, see Chapter 3, Note 5.
3. Apesoa-Varano, "Not Merely TLC"; and Bolton, "Changing Faces." See also Bull and FitzGerald, "Nursing," on the intersection of caring and technology in an operating room setting.
4. Nelson and Gordon, *Complexities of Care*, 13–29.
5. See Apesoa-Varano, "Educated Caring."

6. See Finn, "Language of Teamwork," for a concurring argument.

7. Barlett and Steele, "Critical Condition"; Hacker, *Divided Welfare State*, 221–73; Hacker, "Historical Logic"; Waitzkin, *Second Sickness*; and Waitzkin and Waterman, *Exploitation of Illness*.

8. Bazzoli, "Corporatization of American Hospitals"; and Clark et al., "Healthcare Reform."

9. Bauman and Silverman, "De-Professionalization in Health Care." On the impact of the new managerialism on nursing, see Beardwood et al., "Complaints against Nurses," and Wong, "Caring Holistically." Regarding social work, see Harlow, "New Managerialism." For a more general critique, see Clarke, "Doing the Right Thing?"

10. Wright, "Francis Report." For Weber's discussion of the "iron cage," see *Protestant Ethic*, 181–82.

11. In addition to Freidson, *Professional Dominance*, and Starr, *Social Transformation*, see the more recently published Rodwin, *Conflicts of Interest*.

12. DiPrete, "Upgrading and Downgrading"; Hafferty and Light, "Professional Dynamics"; Hugman, "Social Work and De-professionalization"; Wagner, "Proletarianization of Nursing"; and Wolinsky, "Professional Dominance."

13. Hugman, "Social Work and De-professionalization"; see also Healy and Meagher, "Reprofessionalization of Social Work." On general practitioners, see Pickard, "Professionalization of General Practitioners"; for a similar argument, see also DiPrete, "Upgrading and Downgrading."

14. Freidson, *Professionalism*; see also Hafferty, "Professionalism."

15. C. Davies, "New Vision of Professionalism"; and Salvage, "Rethinking Professionalism."

16. Salvage, "Rethinking Professionalism," 17–18. An extended quote from Salvage (18–19) best summarizes what the new professionalism entails in the context of what I have argued in this book: "Perhaps, then, all health care practitioners should aspire to this plurality—but what of the notion of mastery of their own domain? Even in one closely defined field, this is already impossible with the explosion of information and its accessibility via various media including the Internet. That explosion is also itself breaking down barriers between domains and emphasizing interconnections rather than narrow specialisation. The best a professional can do is learn at the outset how to learn, and commit to a lifelong learning process. Their domain or area of specialisation might change with time, as they become interested in a new challenge or develop new insights and skills, so the work setting needs to encourage and support this flexibility. At the very least all professionals need to be aware of the importance of the plurality of knowledges, and confident enough of their own contribution and its limitations to allow for 'adjustment and negotiation.' There are also some basic skills and knowledge nearly all should possess regardless, such as communication skills, basic life support and nutrition. This points to an education structure and process built around a common core, so that everyone understands and values the differ-

ent knowledges before choosing their own area of specialisation and developing their own particular strengths. It also points to a novice-to-expert ladder that is not profession-specific, so the apprentice doctor can learn from the physio-therapist or the medical consultant mentor the nursing student—if indeed those old professional roles will continue to be viable or desirable. Once knowledge has been reconceptualised, Davies argues, 'surrounding social relations can be transformed.' Decision-making becomes interdependent, with what the patient, carer, nurse and others know and understand of the patient's condition and context ascribed as much value as what the doctor knows. Today, what is called teamwork is often no more than a group of individuals working harmoniously but independently alongside each other. This vision regenerates teamwork as a truly collective endeavour."

Bibliography

Abbott, Andrew. *The System of Professions: An Essay on the Division of Expert Labor.* Chicago: University of Chicago Press, 1988.

———. "Things of Boundaries." *Social Research* 62, no. 4 (1995): 857–82.

Abbott, Pamela, and Liz Meerabeau, eds. *The Sociology of the Caring Professions.* 2nd ed. New York: Routledge, 1998.

Agency for Healthcare Research and Quality. *National Healthcare Disparities Report, 2008.* AHRQ Publication No. 09-0002. Rockville, MD: U.S. Department of Health and Human Services, 2009.

Albert, Tanya. "More Doctors Following Trend to Unionize." *American Medical News* 43, no. 44 (2000): 1–2, 4.

Aldridge, Meryl. "Unlimited Liability? Emotional Labour in Nursing and Social Work." *Journal of Advanced Nursing* 20, no. 4 (1994): 722–28.

Allen, Davina. *The Changing Shape of Nursing Practice: The Role of Nurses in the Hospital Division of Labor.* London: Routledge, 2001.

———. "Doctor-Nurse Relationships: Accomplishing the Skill Mix in Health Care." In Abbott and Meerabeau, *Sociology,* 210–33.

———. "Doing Occupational Demarcation: The 'Boundary-Work' of Nurse Managers in a District General Hospital." *Journal of Contemporary Ethnography* 29, no. 3 (2000): 326–56.

———. "Narrating Nursing Jurisdiction: 'Atrocity Stories' and 'Boundary Work.'" *Symbolic Interaction* 24, no. 1 (2001): 75–103.

———. "The Nursing-Medical Boundary: A Negotiated Order?" *Sociology of Health and Illness* 19, no. 4 (1997): 498–520.

———. "Re-reading Nursing and Re-writing Practice: Towards an Empirically Based Reformulation of the Nursing Mandate." *Nursing Inquiry* 11, no. 4 (2004): 271–83.

Allsop, Judith, and Mike Saks. *Regulating the Health Professions.* London: Sage, 2002.

Angelelli, Claudia V., and Patricia Geist-Martin. "Enhancing Culturally Competent Health Communication: Constructing Understanding between Providers and Culturally Diverse Patients." In Ray, *Health Communication in Practice,* 271–84.

Anspach, Renee R. *Deciding Who Lives: Fateful Choices in the Intensive-Care Nursery.* Berkeley: University of California Press, 1993.

Apesoa-Varano, Ester Carolina. "Educated Caring: The Emergence of Professional Ideology among Nurses." *Qualitative Sociology* 30, no. 3 (2007): 249–74.

———. "Not Merely TLC: Nurses' Caring Skills Revisited." Unpublished manuscript.

Apesoa-Varano, Ester Carolina, Judith C. Barker, and Ladson Hinton. "Curing and

Caring: The Work of Primary Care Physicians with Dementia Patients." *Qualitative Heath Research* 21, no. 11 (2011): 1469–83.

Ashcroft, Richard E. "Current Epistemological Problems in Evidence-Based Medicine." *Journal of Medical Ethics* 30, no. 2 (2004): 131–35.

Barlett, Donald L., and James B. Steele. "Critical Condition: How Healthcare in America Became Big Business and Bad Medicine." In Perrucci and Perrucci, *Transformation of Work*, 593–604.

Baumann, Andrea, and Barbara Silverman. "The De-Professionalization in Health Care: Flattening the Hierarchy." In *The Ethics of the New Economy: Restructuring and Beyond*, edited by Leo Groarke, 203–10. Waterloo, ON: Wilfrid Laurier University Press, 1998.

Bazzoli, Gloria J. "Changes in Resident Physicians' Collective Bargaining Outcomes as Union Strength Declines." *Medical Care* 26, no. 3 (1988): 263–77.

———. "The Corporatization of American Hospitals." *Journal of Health Politics, Policy and Law* 29, no. 4–5 (2004): 885–906.

Beardwood, Barbara. "The Loosening of Professional Boundaries and Restructuring: The Implications for Nursing and Medicine in Ontario, Canada." *Law and Policy* 21, no. 3 (1992): 315–43.

Beardwood, Barbara, Vivienne Walters, John Eyles, and Susan French. "Complaints against Nurses: A Reflection of 'The New Managerialism' and Consumerism in Health Care?" *Social Science and Medicine* 48, no. 3 (1999): 363–74.

Beauchamp, Tom, and James Childress. *Principles of Biomedical Ethics*. New York: Oxford University Press, 2001.

Becker, Howard S., Blanche Geer, Everett C. Hughes, and Anselm L. Strauss. *Boys in White: Student Culture in Medical School*. Chicago: University of Chicago Press, 1961.

Beckett, Chris, and Andrew Maynard. *Values and Ethics in Social Work: An Introduction*. London: Sage, 2005.

Beder, Joan. *Hospital Social Work: The Interface of Medicine and Caring*. New York: Routledge, 2006.

Ben-Sira, Zeev, and Miriam Szyf. "Status Inequality in the Social Worker-Nurse Collaboration in Hospitals." *Social Science and Medicine* 34, no. 4 (1992): 365–74.

Berger, Bennett M. *An Essay on Culture: Symbolic Structure and Social Structure*. Berkeley: University of California Press, 1995.

Bishop, Anne H., and John R. Scudder, Jr., eds. *Caring, Curing, Coping: Nurse, Physician, and Patient Relationships*. Tuscaloosa: University of Alabama Press, 1985.

Bolton, Sharon C. "Changing Faces: Nurses as Emotional Jugglers." *Sociology of Health and Illness* 23, no. 1 (2001): 85–100.

Bowden, Peta. *Caring: Gender-Sensitive Ethics*. London: Routledge, 1997.

Bowers, Warner F. *Interpersonal Relationships in the Hospital*. Springfield, IL: Thomas, 1960.

Braithwaite, Dawn O., and Phyllis Japp. "'They Make Us Miserable in the Name of

Helping Us': Communication of Persons with Visible and Invisible Disabilities." In Ray, *Health Communication in Practice*, 171–80.

Brannon, Robert. *Intensifying Care: The Hospital Industry, Professionalization, and the Reorganization of the Nursing Labor Process*. Amityville, NY: Baywood, 2008.

———. "Professionalization and Work Intensification." In Perrucci and Perrucci, *Transformation of Work*, 314–29.

Brodkin Sacks, Karen. *Caring by the Hour: Women, Work and Organizing at Duke Medical Center*. Urbana: University of Illinois Press, 1988.

Brooten, Dorothy, and Mary D. Naylor. "Nurses' Effect on Changing Patient Outcomes." *Journal of Nursing Scholarship* 27, no. 2 (1995): 95–99.

Budd, Susan, and Ursula Sharma. *The Healing Bond: The Practitioner-Patient Relationship and Therapeutic Responsibility*. London: Routledge, 1994.

Budrys, Grace. *When Physicians Join Unions*. Ithaca, NY: Cornell University Press, 1997.

Bull, Rosalind, and Mary FitzGerald. "Nursing in a Technological Environment: Nursing Care in the Operating Room." *International Journal of Nursing Practice* 12 (2006): 3–7.

Burawoy, Michael. *Manufacturing Consent: Changes in the Labor Process under Monopoly Capitalism*. Chicago: University of Chicago Press, 1979.

Burkett, Gary L., and Dorothy E. Kurz. "A Comparison of the Values and Career Orientations of Male and Female Medical Students: Some Unintended Consequences of U.S. Public Policy." *Health Policy and Education* 2, no. 1 (1981): 33–45.

Campbell, Eric G., James Mountford, Russell L. Gruen, Lawrence G. Miller, Paul D. Cleary, and David Blumenthal. "A National Survey of Physician-Industry Relationships." *New England Journal of Medicine* 356, no. 17 (2007): 1742–50.

Caudill, William A. *The Psychiatric Hospital as a Small Society*. Cambridge, MA: Harvard University Press, 1967.

Chambliss, Daniel F. *Beyond Caring: Hospitals, Nurses, and the Social Organization of Ethics*. Chicago: University of Chicago Press, 1996.

Cheung, Robyn B., Linda H. Aiken, Sean P. Clarke, and Douglas M. Sloane. "Nursing Care and Patient Outcomes: International Evidence." *Enfermeria Clinica* 18, no. 1 (2008): 35–40.

Choi, Thomas, Robert F. Allison, and Fred C. Munson. *Governing University Hospitals in a Changing Environment*. Ann Arbor, MI: Health Administration Press, 1986.

Choudhry, Sugit, and Troyen A. Brennan. "Collective Bargaining by Physicians—Labor Law, Antitrust Law, and Organized Medicine." *New England Journal of Medicine* 345, no. 15 (2001): 1141–44.

Clair, Jeffery Michael, and Richard M. Allman. *Sociomedical Perspectives on Patient Care*. Lexington: University Press of Kentucky, 1993.

Clark, Paul F., Darlene A. Clark, David E. Day, and Dennis E. Shea. "Healthcare Reform and the Workplace Experience of Nurses: Implications for Patient Care and Union Organizing." *Industrial and Labor Relations Review* 55, no. 1 (2001): 132–48.

Clarke, John. "Doing the Right Thing? Managerialism and Social Welfare." In Abbott and Meerabeau, *Sociology*, 234–54.

Cohen, Helen A. *The Nurse's Quest for a Professional Identity*. Menlo Park, CA: Addison-Wesley, 1981.

Conrad, Peter, ed. *The Sociology of Health and Illness: Critical Perspectives*. 8th ed. New York: Worth Publishers, 2009.

Cornell, Stephen, and Douglas Hartmann. *Ethnicity and Race: Making Identities in a Changing World*. 2nd ed. Thousand Oaks, CA: Pine Forge Press, 2006.

Crocker, Ruth Hutchinson. *Social Work and Social Order: The Settlement Movement in Two Industrial Cities, 1889–1930*. Urbana: University of Illinois Press, 1992.

Cusick, Anne, and Lynne Adamson. "Professional Accreditation of Occupational Therapy Educational Programs: A Bright or Embattled Future?" *Australian Occupational Therapy Journal* 51 (2004): 133–43.

Daniels, Arlene Kaplan. "Invisible Work." *Social Problems* 34 (1987): 403–15.

D'Antonio, Patricia. *American Nursing: A History of Knowledge, Authority, and the Meaning of Work*. Baltimore: Johns Hopkins University Press, 2010.

Davies, Bronwyn. "Death to Critique and Dissent? The Policies and Practices of New Managerialism and of 'Evidence-Based Practice.'" *Gender and Education* 15, no. 1 (2003): 91–103.

Davies, Celia. "Competence versus Care? Gender and Caring Revisited." *Acta Sociologica* 38, no. 1 (1995): 17–31.

———. *Gender and the Professional Predicament in Nursing*. Buckingham, UK: Open University Press, 1995.

———. "A New Vision of Professionalism." *Nursing Times* 92, no. 46 (1996): 54.

deLamerens-Pratt, Maite, and Gerald S. Golden. "Teamwork in Medical Settings— Hospitals, Clinics, and Communities." In *Teamwork in Human Services: Models and Applications across the Life Span*, edited by Howard G. Garner and Fred P. Orelove, 159–77. Boston: Butterworth-Heinemann, 1994.

Department of Labor. "Gender Gap in Unionization Closing." *Editor's Desk*, January 19, 2001.

Derber, Charles. "Toward a New Theory of Professionals as Workers: Advanced Capitalism and Postindustrial Labor." In *Professionals as Workers: Mental Labor in Advanced Capitalism*, edited by Charles Derber, 193–208. Boston: G. K. Hall, 1982.

de Tocqueville, Alexis. *Democracy in America*. Garden City, NY: Anchor, 1969.

Diamond, Timothy. *Making Gray Gold: Narratives of Nursing Home Care*. Chicago: University of Chicago Press, 1992.

Di Blasi, Zelda, Elaine Harkness, Edzard Ernst, Amanda Georgiou, and Jos Kleijnen. "Influence of Context Effects on Health Outcomes: A Systematic Review." *Lancet* 357, no. 9258 (2001): 757–62.

DiMatteo, M. Robin, and David Dante DiNicola. *Achieving Patient Compliance: The Psychology of the Medical Practitioner's Role*. New York: Pergamon Press, 1982.

Dingwall, Robert. "Problems of Teamwork in Primary Care." In *Teamwork in the*

Personal Social Services and Health Care, edited by Susan Lonsdale, Adrian Webb, and Thomas L. Briggs, 111–37. Syracuse, NY: Syracuse University School of Social Work; London: Personal Social Services Council, 1980.

Dingwall, Robert, and Davina Allen. "The Implications of Healthcare Reforms for the Profession of Nursing." *Nursing Inquiry* 8, no. 2 (2001): 64–74.

DiPrete, Thomas A. "The Upgrading and Downgrading of Occupations: Status Redefinition vs. Deskilling as Alternative Theories of Change." *Social Forces* 66, no. 3 (1988): 725–46.

Dorroh, Thelma Lee. *Between Patient and Health Worker*. New York: McGraw-Hill, 1974.

Ducey, Ariel. *Never Good Enough: Health Care Workers and the False Promise of Job Training*. Ithaca, NY: Cornell University Press, 2009.

Ehrenreich, Barbara, and John Ehrenreich. "The Professional-Managerial Class." In *Between Labor and Capital*, edited by Pat Walker, 4–45. Boston: South End Press, 1979.

Ehrenreich, John. *The Altruistic Imagination: A History of Social Work and Social Policy in the United States*. Ithaca, NY: Cornell University Press, 1985.

Emerick, Lon L. *The Client-Clinician Relationship: Essays on Interpersonal Sensitivity in the Therapeutic Transaction*. Springfield, IL: Thomas, 1974.

England, Paula, Michelle Budig, and Nancy Folbre. "Wages of Virtue: The Relative Pay of Care Work." *Social Problems* 49, no. 4 (2002): 455–73.

Epstein, Cynthia Fuchs. *Deceptive Distinctions: Sex, Gender and the Social Order*. New York: Russell Sage Foundation, 1988.

———. "Tinkerbells and Pinups: The Construction of Gender Boundaries at Work." In *Cultivating Differences: Symbolic Boundaries and the Making of Inequality*, edited by Michelle Lamont and Marcel Fournier, 232–56. Chicago: University of Chicago Press, 1992.

Etzioni, Amitai. *The Semi-Professions and Their Organization: Teachers, Nurses, and Social Workers*. New York: Free Press, 1969.

Fagerhaugh, Shizuko Y., and Anselm L. Strauss. *Politics of Pain Management: Staff-Patient Interaction*. Menlo Park, CA: Addison-Wesley, 1977.

Fantasia, Rick. *Cultures of Solidarity: Consciousness, Action, and Contemporary American Workers*. Berkeley: University of California Press, 1989.

Feinstein, Alvan R., and Ralph I. Horwitz. "Problems in the 'Evidence' of 'Evidence-Based Medicine.'" *American Journal of Medicine* 103, no. 6 (1997): 529–35.

Finch, Janet, and Dulcie Groves, eds. *A Labour of Love: Women, Work, and Caring*. London: Routledge, 1983.

Finch, J. S. "Unionization in Respiratory Therapy." *Respiratory Therapy* 5, no. 4 (1975): 12–72.

Finn, Rachael. "The Language of Teamwork: Reproducing Professional Divisions in the Operating Theatre." *Human Relations* 61, no. 1 (2008): 103–30.

Finn, Rachael, Mark Learmonth, and Patrick Reedy. "Some Unintended Effects of Teamwork in Healthcare." *Social Science and Medicine* 70, no. 8 (2010): 1148–54.

Folbre, Nancy, ed. *For Love and Money: Care Provision in the United States*. New York: Russell Sage Foundation, 2012.

———. *The Invisible Heart: Economics and Family Values*. New York: New Press, 2001.

Foley, Laura, and Christopher A. Faircloth. "Medicine as Discursive Resource: Legitimation in the Work Narratives of Midwives." *Sociology of Health and Illness* 25, no. 2 (2003): 165–84.

Foner, Nancy. *The Caregiving Dilemma: Work in an American Nursing Home*. Berkeley: University of California Press, 1994.

Ford, Leigh Arden, and Brigitte Cobbs Christmon. "'Every Breast Cancer Is Different': Illness Narratives and the Management of Identity in Breast Cancer." In Ray, *Health Communication in Practice*, 157–70.

Francis, Robert, chair. *Report of the Mid Staffordshire NHS Foundation Trust Public Inquiry* [the "Francis Report"]. Norwich, UK: Stationery Office, 2013. Available at *www.midstaffspublicinquiry.com*.

Freidson, Eliot, ed. *The Hospital in Modern Society*. London: Free Press of Glencoe, 1963.

———. *Professional Dominance: The Social Structure of Medical Care*. New York: Atherton Press, 1970.

———. *Professionalism: The Third Logic*. Cambridge: Polity Press, 2001.

———. *Profession of Medicine: A Study of the Sociology of Applied Knowledge*. New York: Dodd, Mead, 1970.

Friedman, Howard, and M. Robin DiMatteo. *Interpersonal Issues in Health Care*. New York: Academic Press, 1982.

Friedman, Marilyn. "Beyond Caring: The De-Moralization of Gender." *Canadian Journal of Philosophy* 13, supplement (1987): 87–110.

Gans, Herbert J. *The Urban Villagers: Group and Class in the Life of Italian-Americans*. New York: Free Press, 1982.

———. *The War against the Poor: The Underclass and Antipoverty Policy*. New York: Basic Books, 1995.

Garman, Andrew N., David C. Leach, and Nancy Spector. "Worldviews in Collision: Conflict and Collaboration across Professional Lines." *Journal of Organizational Behavior* 27, no. 7 (2006): 829–49.

Garson, Barbara. *All the Livelong Day: The Meaning and Demeaning of Routine Work*. New York: Penguin, 1994.

Gawande, Atul. *Better: A Surgeon's Notes on Performance*. New York: Metropolitan, 2007.

———. "Personal Best: Top Athletes and Singers Have Coaches. Should You?" *New Yorker*, October 3, 2011, *www.newyorker.com*.

Gerson, Judith, and Katy Peiss. "Boundaries, Negotiations, Consciousness: Reconceptualizing Gender Relations." *Social Problems* 32 (1985): 317–31.

Gieryn, Thomas F. "Boundary Work and the Demarcation of Science from Non-Science: Strains and Interests in the Professional Ideologies of Scientists." *American Sociological Review* 48, no. 6 (1983): 781–95.

Glomb, Theresa M., John Kammeyer-Mueller, and Mary Rotundo. "Emotional Labor Demands and Compensating Wage Differentials." *Journal of Applied Psychology* 89, no. 4 (2004): 700–14.

Goffman, Erving. *Asylums: Essays on the Social Situation of Mental Patients and Other Inmates*. Garden City, NY: Anchor, 1961.

———. *Interaction Ritual: Essays in Face-to-Face Behavior*. Chicago: Aldine, 1967.

Goldsmith, Jeff C. *Can Hospitals Survive? The New Competitive Health Care Market*. Homewood, IL: Dow Jones-Irwin, 1981.

Goodman-Draper, Jacqueline. *Health Care's Forgotten Majority: Nurses and Their Frayed White Collars*. Westport, CT: Auburn House, 1995.

Gouldner, Alvin W. *The Future of Intellectuals and the Rise of the New Class*. New York: Oxford University Press, 1979.

Graham, Hilary. "Caring: Labour of Love." In Finch and Groves, *Labour of Love*, 13–30.

Griffin, Donald J., ed. *Hospitals: What They Are and How They Work*. 4th ed. Sudbury, MA: Jones and Bartlett Learning, 2012.

Groopman, Jerome. "Doctors and Patients: A Great Case." *New England Journal of Medicine* 351, no. 20 (2004): 2043–45.

———. *How Doctors Think*. Boston: Houghton Mifflin, 2007.

———. *Second Opinions: Stories of Intuition and Choice in the Changing World of Medicine*. New York: Viking, 2000.

Gruen, Russell L., Eric G. Campbell, and David Blumenthal. "Public Roles of US Physicians: Community Participation, Political Involvement, and Collective Advocacy." *JAMA: The Journal of the American Medical Association* 296, no. 20 (2006): 2467–75.

Guadagnino, Christopher. "Physician Unions Gain Steam." *Physician's News Digest*, December 1997, *www.physiciansnews.com*.

Hacker, Jacob S. *The Divided Welfare State: The Battle over Public and Private Social Benefits in the United States*. New York: Cambridge University Press, 2002.

———. "The Historical Logic of National Health Insurance: Structure and Sequence in the Development of British, Canadian, and U.S. Medical Policy." *Studies in American Political Development* 12, no. 1 (1998): 57–130.

Hafferty, Frederic W. "Professionalism: The Next Wave." *New England Journal of Medicine* 355, no. 20 (2006): 2151–52.

Hafferty, Frederic W., and Donald W. Light. "Professional Dynamics and the Changing Nature of Medical Work." *Journal of Health and Social Behavior* 35 (1995): 132–53.

Halpern, Sydney A. "Dynamics of Professional Control: Internal Coalitions and Crossprofessional Boundaries." *American Journal of Sociology* 97, no. 4 (1992): 994–1021.

Harlow, Elizabeth. "New Managerialism, Social Service Departments, and Social Work Practice Today." *Practice: Social Work in Action* 15, no. 2 (2003): 29–44.

Harrington Meyer, Madonna. *Care Work: Gender, Labor, and the Welfare State*. New York: Routledge, 2000.

Hartley, Heather. "The System of Alignments Challenging Professional Dominance: An Elaborated Theory of Countervailing Powers." *Sociology of Health and Illness* 24, no. 2 (2002): 178–207.

Harvey, Janet. "Up-Skilling and the Intensification of Work: The 'Extended Role' in Intensive Care Nursing and Midwifery." *Sociological Review* 43, no. 4 (1995): 765–81.

Haskell, Thomas L. *The Authority of Experts: Studies in History and Theory*. Bloomington: Indiana University Press, 1984.

Haynes, John H. "The 'Rank and File Movement' in Private Social Work." *Labor History* 16, no. 1 (1975): 78–98.

Health Resources and Services Administration. *The Registered Nurse Population: Findings from the March 2004 National Sample Survey of Registered Nurses*. Rockville, MD: U.S. Department of Health and Human Services, 2006. *bhpr.hrsa.gov /healthworkforce/rnsurveys/rnsurvey2004.pdf.*

Health Resources and Services Administration. *The Registered Nurse Population: Findings from the 2008 National Sample Survey of Registered Nurses*. Rockville, MD: U.S. Department of Health and Human Services, 2010. *bhpr.hrsa.gov /healthworkforce/rnsurvey2008.html.*

Healy, Karen, and Gabrielle Meagher. "The Reprofessionalization of Social Work: Collaborative Approaches for Achieving Professional Recognition." *British Journal of Social Work* 34, no. 2 (2004): 243–60.

Held, Virginia. *The Ethics of Care: Personal, Political, and Global*. Oxford: Oxford University Press, 2006.

Heritage, John, and Douglas W. Maynard. *Communication in Medical Care: Interaction between Primary Care Physicians and Patients*. Cambridge: Cambridge University Press, 2006.

Hinz, Christine A. *Communicating with Patients: Skills for Building Rapport*. Chicago: American Medical Association, 2000.

Hochschild, Arlie Russell. *The Managed Heart: Commercialization of Human Feeling*. Berkeley: University of California Press, 1983.

Hodson, Randy. "Worker Resistance: An Underdeveloped Concept in the Sociology of Work." *Economic and Industrial Democracy* 16, no. 79 (1995): 79–110.

Hoff, Timothy J. "Physician Unionization in the United States: Fad or Phenomenon?" *Journal of Health and Human Services Administration* 23, no. 1 (2000): 5–23.

Hollingsworth, Joseph Rogers, and Ellen Jane Hollingsworth. *Controversy about American Hospitals: Funding, Ownership, and Performance*. Washington, DC: American Enterprise Institute for Public Policy Research, 1987.

Howard, Jan, and Anselm Strauss. *Humanizing Health Care*. New York: Wiley, 1975.

Hughes, David. "When Nurse Knows Best: Some Aspects of Nurse/Doctor Interaction in a Casualty Department." *Sociology of Health and Illness* 10, no. 1 (1988): 1–22.

Hugman, Richard. *New Approaches in the Ethics for the Caring Professions.* New York: Palgrave Macmillan, 2005.

——. "Social Work and De-professionalization." In Abbott and Meerabeau, *Sociology,* 178–98.

Hurwitz, Brian, Trisha Greenhalgh, and Vieda Skultans, eds. *Narrative Research in Health and Illness.* Malden, MA: BMJ Books/Blackwell Publishing, 2004.

Hwang, Lucia. "Ratio Roundup." *California Nurse: The Official Bulletin of the California Nurses Association,* January/February 2005, 6–7.

Institute of Medicine. *The Future of Nursing: Leading Change, Advancing Health.* Washington, DC: National Academies Press, 2010. *www.iom.edu/reports.*

Jacobs, Jerry A., and Ann K. Boulis. *The Changing Face of Medicine: Women Doctors and the Evolution of Health Care in America.* Ithaca, NY: Cornell University Press, 2008.

Jacobs, Jerry A., and Kathleen Gerson. *The Time Divide: Work, Family, and Gender Inequality.* Cambridge, MA: Harvard University Press, 2004.

Jacobs, Linda A., Mary Jane K. DiMattio, Sheldon D. Fields, and Tammi L. Bishop. "The Baccalaureate Degree in Nursing as an Entry-Level Requirement for Professional Nursing Practice." *Journal of Professional Nursing* 14, no. 4 (1998): 225–33.

Kaplan, Sherrie H., Sheldon Greenfield, and John E. Ware, Jr. "Assessing the Effects of Physician-Patient Interactions on the Outcomes of Chronic Disease." *Medical Care* 27, no. 3 (1989): S110.

Keller, Evelyn Fox. *Making Sense of Life: Explaining Biological Development with Models, Metaphors, and Machines.* Cambridge, MA: Harvard University Press, 2003.

Keller, Evelyn Fox, and Helen E. Longino. *Feminism and Science.* Oxford: Oxford University Press, 1996.

Kemp, Donna R. *Mental Health in America: A Reference Book.* Santa Barbara, CA: ABC-CLIO, 2007.

Kimball, Bruce A. *The "True Professional Ideal" in America: A History.* Oxford: Blackwell, 1992.

Kunzel, Regina G. *Fallen Women, Problem Girls: Unmarried Mothers and the Professionalization of Social Work, 1890–1945.* New Haven, CT: Yale University Press, 1993.

Lamont, Michelle. *Money, Morals, and Manners: The Culture of the French and the American Upper-Middle Class.* Chicago: University of Chicago Press, 1992.

Lamont, Michelle, and Virag Molnar. "The Study of Boundaries in the Social Sciences." *Annual Review of Sociology* 28 (2002): 167–95.

Larkin, Gerald V. "Medical Dominance and Control: Radiographers in the Division of Labour." *Sociological Review* 26, no. 4 (1978): 843–58.

Larson, Eric B., and Xin Yao. "Clinical Empathy as Emotional Labor in the Patient-Physician Relationship." *JAMA: The Journal of the American Medical Association* 293, no. 9 (2005): 1100–1106.

Larson, Magali Sarfatti. *The Rise of Professionalism: A Sociological Analysis.* Berkeley: University of California Press, 1977.

Leander, William J., Dennis L. Shortridge, and Phyllis M. Watson. *Patients First: Experiences of a Patient-Focused Pioneer.* Chicago: Health Administration Press, 1996.

Leiby, James. *A History of Social Welfare and Social Work in the United States.* New York: Columbia University Press, 1978.

Leidner, Robin. "Serving Hamburgers and Selling Insurance: Gender, Work, and Identity in Interactive Service Jobs." *Gender and Society* 5, no. 2 (1991): 154–77.

Leighninger, Leslie. *Social Work: Search for Identity.* New York: Greenwood Press, 1987.

Liebow, Elliot. *Tally's Corner: A Study of Negro Streetcorner Men.* Boston: Little, Brown, 1967.

———. *Tell Them Who I Am: The Lives of Homeless Women.* New York: Maxwell Macmillan International, 1993.

Light, Donald W. "Countervailing Power: The Changing Character of the Medical Profession in the United States." In Conrad, *Sociology of Health and Illness*, 239–48.

Light, Donald W., and Sol Levine. "The Changing Character of the Medical Profession: A Theoretical Overview." *Milbank Quarterly* 66 (1988): 10–32.

Lipkin, Gladys B., and Roberta G. Cohen. *Effective Approaches to Patients' Behavior: A Guide Book for Health Care Professionals, Patients, and Their Caregivers.* New York: Springer, 1998.

Lively, Kathryn. "Occupational Claims to Professionalism: The Case of Paralegals." *Symbolic Interaction* 24, no. 3 (2001): 343–66.

Lo, Ming-Cheng M., and Clare L. Stacey. "Beyond Cultural Competency: Bourdieu, Patients and Clinical Encounters." *Sociology of Health and Illness* 30, no. 5 (2008): 741–55.

Lopez, Steven H. "Emotional Labor and Organized Emotional Care: Conceptualizing Nursing Home Care Work." *Work and Occupations* 33, no. 2 (2006): 133–60.

Lorber, Judith. "Good Patients, Problem Patients: Conformity and Deviance in a General Hospital." *Journal of Health and Social Behavior* 16, no. 2 (1975): 213–25.

Luepke, Ellen. "White Coat, Blue Collar: Physician Unionization and Managed Care." *Annals of Health Law* 8 (1999): 275–99.

MacCallum, David. "The Case in Social Work: Psychological Assessment and Social Regulation." In Abbott and Meerabeau, *Sociology*, 73–81.

Makary, Marty. *Unaccountable: What Hospitals Won't Tell You and How Transparency Can Revolutionize Health Care.* New York: Bloomsbury Press, 2012.

Manthey, Marie. *The Practice of Primary Nursing.* Boston: Blackwell Scientific Publications, 1980.

Martin, John. *Hospitals in Trouble.* Oxford: Blackwell, 1984.

McKinlay, John B., and Lisa D. Marceau. "The End of the Golden Age of Doctoring." *International Journal of Health Services* 32, no. 2 (2002): 379–416.

McMurtry, Dana Elbein. *Hospital Nursing in the '90s: The Effect on Patient Care.* Chicago, IL: American Hospital Association, 1991.

Mechanic, David. *Mental Health and Social Policy: The Emergence of Managed Care.* Boston: Allyn and Bacon, 1999.

———. *The Truth about Health Care: Why Reform Is Not Working in America*. New Brunswick, NJ: Rutgers University Press, 2006.

Melia, Kath. *Learning and Working: The Occupational Socialization of Nurses*. London: Tavistock, 1987.

———. "Student Nurses' Construction of Occupational Socialization." *Sociology of Health and Illness* 6, no. 2 (1984): 132–51.

Melosh, Barbara. "'Not Merely a Profession': Nurses and Resistance to Professionalization." *American Behavioral Scientist* 32, no. 6 (1989): 668–79.

———. *"The Physician's Hand": Work Culture and Conflict in American Nursing*. Philadelphia: Temple University Press, 1982.

Merton, Robert. *Social Theory and Social Structure*. Glencoe, IL: Free Press, 1957.

Mesler, Mark A. "Boundary Encroachment and Task Delegation: Clinical Pharmacists on the Medical Team." *Sociology of Health and Illness* 13, no. 3 (1991): 310–31.

Mishoe, Shelley C. "Current and Future Credentialing in Respiratory Therapy." *Respiratory Care* 25, no. 3 (1980): 345–52.

Mitchell, Gail J. "Evidence-Based Practice: Critique and Alternative View." *Nursing Science Quarterly* 12, no. 1 (1999): 30–35.

Moberg, David. "Nurses Fight to Retain Right to Unionize." *In These Times*, August 2006, 8–9.

Moffat, Marilyn. "The History of Physical Therapy Practice in the United States." *Journal of Physical Therapy Education* 17, no. 3 (2004): 15–25.

Muff, Janet. *Socialization, Sexism, and Stereotyping: Women's Issues in Nursing*. Toronto: Mosby, 1982.

Myerscough, Philip R., and Michael J. Ford. *Talking with Patients: Keys to Good Communication*. Oxford: Oxford University Press, 1996.

Mykhalovskiy, Eric, and Lorna Weir. "The Problem of Evidence-Based Medicine: Directions for Social Science." *Social Science and Medicine* 59, no. 5 (2004): 1059–69.

Nam, Charles B., and Monica Boyd. "Occupational Status in 2000: Over a Century of Census-Based Measurement." *Population Research and Policy Review* 23, no 4 (2004): 327–58.

Neil, Ruth M., and Robin Watts. *Caring and Nursing: Explorations in Feminist Perspectives*. New York: National League for Nursing, 1991.

Nelson, Sioban, and Suzanne Gordon. *The Complexities of Care: Nursing Reconsidered*. Ithaca, NY: Cornell University Press, 2006.

Noddings, Nel. *Caring: A Feminine Approach to Ethics and Moral Education*. Berkeley: University of California Press, 1984.

———. *The Challenge to Care in Schools: An Alternative Approach to Education*. New York: Teachers College Press, 2005.

Norris, Pauline. "How 'We' Are Different from 'Them': Occupational Boundary Maintenance in the Treatment of Musculo-skeletal Problems." *Sociology of Health and Illness* 23, no. 1 (2001): 24–43.

Parker, Mike, and Jane Slaughter. *Choosing Sides: Unions and the Team Concept*. Boston: South End Press, 1988.

Patterson, Brandy R., Kristopher J. Kimball, Julie B. Walsh-Covarrubias, and Larry
    C. Kilgore. "Effecting the Sixth Core Competency: A Project-Based Curriculum."
    American Journal of Obstetrics and Gynecology 199, no. 5 (2008): 561.e1-561.e6.
Peabody, Francis W. *Doctor and Patient: Papers on the Relationship between the Physi-
    cian to Men and Institutions.* New York: Macmillan, 1930.
Perrucci, Robert, and Carolyn C. Perrucci, eds. *The Transformation of Work in the
    New Economy.* Los Angeles: Roxbury Publishing, 2007.
Peters, Christine. *Powerful Occupational Therapists: A Community of Professionals,
    1950–1980.* New York: Routledge, 2012.
Pickard, Susan. "The Professionalization of General Practitioners with a Special Inter-
    est: Rationalization, Restratification, and Governmentality." *Sociology* 43, no. 2
    (2009): 250–67.
Porter, Sam. "A Participant Observation Study of Power Relations between Nurses
    and Doctors in a General Hospital." *Journal of Advanced Nursing* 16, no. 1 (1991):
    728–35.
Ray, Eileen Berlin, ed. *Health Communication in Practice.* London: Erlbaum Associ-
    ates, 2005.
Reskin, Barbara F., and Patricia A. Roos. *Job Queues, Gender Queues: Explaining
    Women's Inroads into Male Occupations.* Philadelphia: Temple University Press,
    1990.
Reverby, Susan M. *Ordered to Care: The Dilemma of American Nursing, 1850–1945.*
    Cambridge: Cambridge University Press, 1987.
Rintamaki, Lance S., and Dale E. Brashers. "Social Identity and Stigma Management
    for People Living with HIV." In Ray, *Health Communication in Practice*, 145–56.
Riska, Elianne. "Towards Gender Balance: But Will Women Physicians Have an Impact
    on Medicine?" *Social Science and Medicine* 52, no. 2 (2001): 179–87.
Rodwin, Marc A. *Conflicts of Interest and the Future of Medicine: The United States,
    France, and Japan.* New York: Oxford University Press, 2011.
———. *Medicine, Money, and Morals: Physicians' Conflicts of Interests.* New York:
    Oxford University Press, 1993.
Royal College of Physicians. *Doctors in Society: Medical Professionalism in a Changing
    World.* London: Royal College of Physicians, 2005.
Russell, Raymond. *Sharing Ownership in the Workplace.* Albany: State University of
    New York Press, 1985.
Sackett, David L., William M. Rosenberg, J. A. Muir Gray, R. Brian Haynes, and W.
    Scott Richardson. "Evidence Based Medicine: What It Is and What It Isn't." *BMJ:
    British Medical Journal* 312, no. 7023 (1996): 71.
Saks, Mike. *Professions and the Public Interest: Medical Power, Altruism, and Alterna-
    tive Medicine.* London: Routledge, 1995.
Salamon, Julie. *Hospital: Man, Woman, Birth, Death, Infinity, Plus Red Tape, Bad Be-
    havior, Money, God, and Diversity on Steroids.* New York: Penguin, 2008.
Salvage, Jane. "Rethinking Professionalism: The First Step for Patient-Focused Care?"

White paper, Future Health Worker Project, Institute of Public Policy Research, London, 2002.

Schuhmann, Thomas M. "Hospital Financial Performance Trends to Watch." *Healthcare Financial Management* 62, no. 7 (2008): 59–66.

Schur, Lisa A., and Douglas L. Kruse. "Gender Differences in Attitudes toward Unions." *Industrial and Labor Relations Review* 46, no. 1 (1992): 89–102.

Shanafelt, Tait D., Sonja Boone, Litjen Tan, Lotte N. Dyrbye, Wayne Sotile, Daniel Satele, Colin P. West, Jeff Sloan, and Michael R. Oreskovich. "Burnout and Satisfaction with Work-Life Balance among US Physicians Relative to the General US Population." *Archives of Internal Medicine* 172, no. 18 (2012): 1377–85.

Shelledy, David C., and Carl P. Wiezalis. "Education and Credentialing in Respiratory Therapy: Where Are We and Where Should We Be Headed?" *Respiratory Care Clinics of North America* 11, no. 3 (2005): 517–30.

Sibeon, Roger. "The Construction of a Contemporary Sociology of Social Work." In *The Sociology of Social Work*, edited by Martin Davies, 17–67. London: Routledge, 1991.

———. "Social Work Knowledge, Social Actors, and Deprofessionalization." In *The Sociology of the Caring Professions*, 1st ed., edited by Pamela Abbott and Claire Wallace. Basingstoke, UK: Falmer, 1990.

Smith, Vicki. *Managing in the Corporate Interest: Control and Resistance in an American Bank*. Berkeley: University of California Press, 1990.

Spano, Rick. *The Rank and File Movement in Social Work*. Washington, DC: University Press of America, 1982.

Stacey, Clare L. *The Caring Self: The Work Experiences of Home Care Aides*. Ithaca, NY: Cornell University Press, 2011.

———. "Labor's Love Learned: Experiences of Home Health Workers Caring for Elderly and Disabled Adults." PhD diss., University of California, Davis, 2004.

Stacey, Margaret. "The Division of Labour Revisited or Overcoming the Two Adams." In *Practice and Progress: British Sociology, 1950-1980*, edited by Phillip Abrams, R. Deem, J. Finch, and P. Rock, 172–90. London: Allen and Unwin, 1981.

Starr, Paul. *The Social Transformation of American Medicine*. New York: Basic Books, 1982.

Stewart, Karen J. "Promoting Professionalism and Reducing Staff Turnover in Respiratory Care." *Respiratory Care* 50, no. 8 (2005): 1029–30.

Stewart, Moira A. "Effective Physician-Patient Communication and Health Outcomes: A Review." *Canadian Medical Association Journal* 152, no. 9 (1995): 1423–33.

Stewart, Moira A., Judith Belle Brown, Allan Donner, Ian R. McWhinney, Julian Oates, W. Wayne Weston, and John Jordan. "The Impact of Patient-Centered Care on Outcomes." *Journal of Family Practice* 49, no. 9 (2000): 796–804.

Strauss, Anselm L. *Medical Ghettos*. Ann Arbor, MI: Radical Education Project, 1967.

———. *Negotiations: Varieties, Contexts, Processes, and Social Order*. San Francisco: Jossey- Bass, 1978.

———. *Psychiatric Ideologies and Institutions*. New York: Free Press of Glencoe, 1964.

———. "Work and the Division of Labor." *Sociological Quarterly* 26, no. 1 (1985): 1–19.

Strauss, Anselm L., Shizuko Fagerhaugh, Barbara Suczek, and Carolyn Wiener. *The Social Organization of Medical Work*. New Brunswick, NJ: Transaction Publishers, 1997.

Strauss, Anselm L., Leonard Schatzman, Danuta Ehrlich, Rue Bucher, and Melvin Sabshin. "The Hospital and Its Negotiated Order." In Freidson, *Hospital in Modern Society*, 147–219.

Sullivan, William M. "What Is Left of Professionalism after Managed Care." *Hastings Center Report* 29, no. 2 (1999): 7–13.

Surbone, Antonella, and Matjaz Zwitter. *Communication with the Cancer Patient: Information and Truth*. New York: New York Academy of Sciences, 1997.

Svensson, Roland. "The Interplay between Doctors and Nurses—A Negotiated Order Perspective." *Sociology of Health and Illness* 18, no. 3 (1996): 379–98.

Sweet, Victoria. *God's Hotel: A Doctor, a Hospital, and a Pilgrimage to the Heart of Medicine*. New York: Riverhead Books, 2012.

Tanner, Judith, and Stephen Timmons. "Backstage in the Theatre." *Journal of Advanced Nursing* 32, no. 4 (2000): 975–80.

Thomas, William I., and Dorothy Swaine Thomas. *The Child in America: Behavior Problems and Programs*. New York: Knopf, 1928.

Thompson, Teresa L., and Catherine Gilloti. "Staying Out of the Line of Fire: A Medical Student Learns about Bad News Delivery." In Ray, *Health Communication in Practice*, 11–26.

Thorne, Barrie. *Gender Play: Girls and Boys in School*. New Brunswick, NJ: Rutgers University Press, 1993.

Timmermans, Stefan, and Aaron Mauck. "The Promises and Pitfalls of Evidence-Based Medicine." *Health Affairs* 24, no. 1 (2005): 18–28.

Timmons, Stephen, and Judith Tanner. "A Disputed Occupational Boundary: Operating Theatre Nurses and Operating Department Practitioners." *Sociology of Health and Illness* 26, no. 5 (2004): 645–66.

Tronto, Joan C. "Care as a Political Concept." In *Revisioning the Political: Feminist Reconstructions of Traditional Concepts in Western Political Theory*, edited by Nancy J. Hirschmann and Christine Di Stefano, 139–56. Boulder: Westview Press, 1996.

———. *Moral Boundaries: A Political Argument for an Ethic of Care*. New York: Routledge, 1993.

Ungerson, Clare. *Gender and Caring: Work and Welfare in Britain and Scandinavia*. London: Harvester Wheatsheaf, 1990.

———. "Why Do Women Care?" In Finch and Groves, *Labour of Love*, 31–49.

Unland, James. "Physician Unions: Bad for Them and Us." *Physician's News Digest*, March 1997, *www.physiciansnews.com*.

Van Servellen, Gwen. *Communication Skills for the Health Care Professional: Concepts and Techniques*. Sudbury, MA: Jones and Bartlett Learning, 1997.

Varano, Charles. *Forced Choices: Class, Community, and Worker Ownership.* Albany: State University of New York Press, 1999.

Waerness, Kari. "The Rationality of Caring." *Economic and Industrial Democracy* 5 (1984): 185–211.

Wagner, David. "The Proletarianization of Nursing in the United States, 1932–1946." *International Journal of Health Services* 10, no. 2 (1980): 271–90.

Wailoo, Keith, Timothy Stoltzfus Jost, and Mark Schlesinger. "Professional Sovereignty in a Changing Health Care System: Reflections on Paul Starr's *The Social Transformation of American Medicine." Journal of Health Politics, Policy and Law* 29, nos. 4–5 (2004): 557–68.

Waitzkin, Howard. *The Second Sickness: Contradictions of Capitalist Health Care.* Lanham, MD: Rowman and Littlefield, 2000.

Waitzkin, Howard, and Barbara Waterman. *The Exploitation of Illness in Capitalist Society.* Indianapolis: Bobbs-Merrill, 1974.

Walkowitz, Daniel J. *Working with Class: Social Workers and the Politics of Middle-Class Identity.* Chapel Hill: University of North Carolina Press, 1999.

Wallace, Samuel E. *Total Institutions.* Chicago: Aldine, 1971.

Wallis, M. A. "Profession and Professionalism and the Emerging Profession of Occupational Therapy: Part 1." *British Journal of Occupational Therapy* 50, no. 8 (1987): 264–65.

———. "Profession and Professionalism and the Emerging Profession of Occupational Therapy: Part 2." *British Journal of Occupational Therapy* 50, no. 8 (1987): 300–302.

Weber, Max. *The Protestant Ethic and the Spirit of Capitalism.* New York: Scribner, 1958.

Weinberg, Dana B. *Code Green: Money-Driven Hospitals and the Dismantling of Nursing.* Ithaca, NY: Cornell University Press, 2003.

Wenocur, Stanley, and Michael Reisch. *From Charity to Enterprise: The Development of American Social Work in a Market Economy.* Urbana: University of Illinois Press, 1989.

Wicks, Deidre. *Nurses and Doctors at Work: Rethinking Professional Boundaries.* Buckingham, UK: Open University Press, 1998.

Wilkerson, John D. "The Political Economy of Health in the United States." *Annual Review of Political Science* 6, no. 1 (2003): 327–43.

Williams, Christine L. *Still a Man's World: Men Who Do "Women's Work."* Berkeley: University of California Press, 1995.

Williams, Jan. "What Is a Profession? Experience versus Expertise." In *Health, Welfare, and Practice: Reflecting on Roles and Relationships,* edited by Jan Walmsley, Jill Reynolds, Pam Shakespeare, and Ray Wolfe. London: Sage, 1993.

Witz, Anne. *Professions and Patriarchy.* London: Routledge, 1992.

Wolinsky, Fredric D. "The Professional Dominance, Deprofessionalization, Proletarianization and Corporatization Perspectives: An Overview and Synthesis." In *The Changing Medical Profession: An International Perspective,* edited by Frederic W. Hafferty and John B. McKinlay, 11–24. Oxford: Oxford University Press, 1993.

Wolinsky, Howard, and Tom Brune. *The Serpent on the Staff: The Unhealthy Politics of the American Medical Association*. New York: Putnam, 1994.

Wong, Woon Hau. "Caring Holistically within New Managerialism." *Nursing Inquiry* 11, no. 1 (2004): 2–13.

Wright, Oliver. "The Francis Report: Key Findings." *Independent* (London), February 6, 2013. *www.independent.co.uk*.

Zuboff, Shoshana. *In the Age of the Smart Machine: The Future of Work and Power*. New York: Basic Books, 1988.

Zugar, Abigail. "Dissatisfaction with Medical Practice." *New England Journal of Medicine* 350, no. 1 (2004): 69–75.

Zussman, Robert. *Intensive Care: Medical Ethics and the Medical Profession*. Chicago: University of Chicago Press, 1992.

Index